WHAT COLOUR IS YOUR BUILDING?

Measuring and reducing the energy and carbon footprint of buildings

David H. Clark

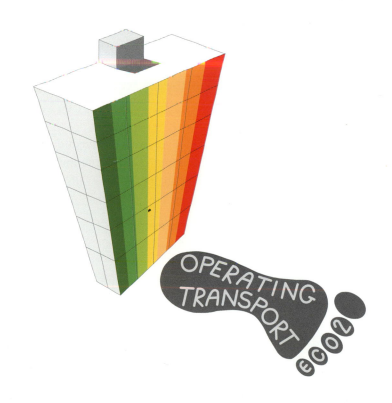

RIBA 🏛 **Publishing**

'What Colour Is Your Building? is an important and timely guide to help us navigate the often misunderstood subject of energy use in and around buildings. Debunking myths and providing a simple step by step guide to measuring and minimising real energy use, this is essential reading.'

PAUL KING
CEO of UK Green Building Council

'David is one of our leading exponents of low energy buildings. I commend this work to designers and contractors, as an embodiment of professional expertise, scholarly insight and remarkable common sense.'

ANDREW MCNAUGHTON
CEO Balfour Beatty plc
and Vice President of the Institution of Civil Engineers

'Rooted in evidence, tempered by experience, and focussed on performance, What Colour Is Your Building? is an indispensable read for anyone who is serious about tackling carbon emissions. The ideas presented by David Clark are original, actionable, commendable and ultimately profitable. We can only hope that more practitioners follow his example and that more decision-makers heed this advice.'

RICHARD FRANCIS
Director of Environment & Sustainability at Gardiner & Theobald
and Chair of BCSC Low Carbon Working Group.

'This book clearly sets out the importance of considering buildings in the round, as a whole system. I'd make this compulsory reading for all 'built environment' students and certainly would encourage all practitioners with an interest in the sustainability of buildings to put it at the top of their reading lists.'

MILES KEEPING
Partner of Deloitte Real Estate and
Chairman of Investment Property Forum Sustainability Interest Group

'What Colour is Your Building? offers a rare combination of asking the right questions and providing detailed answers and is essential reading for all sustainable construction and property practitioners.'

STEVEN BORNCAMP
co-Director of Construction21: International,
Managing Director of Living Future Europe and
Founding President of Romania Green Building Council

'This is a timely and very significant work, one of the first to look comprehensively at the energy and carbon impacts of buildings in their totality. Guidance and data is clearly presented and in a straightforward way free from jargon. I would commend it highly to practitioners, clients and researchers alike.'

PROFESSOR JOHN CONNAUGHTON

University of Reading, School of Construction Management and Engineering

'This lucid and comprehensive book demonstrates that lower environmental impacts – critically the reduction of carbon dioxide emissions – can be achieved through design strategies based on a sound understanding of actual building performance. Its message is that the requisite knowledge isn't rocket science; it requires scientific rigour and design innovation for sure, but common sense and objectivity are the primary requirements for the green buildings of the future.'

RAB BENNETTS, OBE

Director, Bennetts Associates

'Data presented clearly, and with a touch of humour, make this a very good and timely read. The industry has been learning a lot about how to – and how not to – design, construct and manage green buildings. David's book is a concise, accessible summary of the lessons.'

POORAN DESAI, OBE

co-founder BioRegional and International Director,
One Planet Communities

'Real performance is tied to better metrics and more transparency across every dimension – energy, of course, but also water, waste, and materials. David's call to action rings true for anyone who sees better buildings and communities as the cornerstones for a better future.'

S. RICHARD FEDRIZZI

Chairman of World Green Building Council and
President, CEO & Founding Chair of U.S. Green Building Council

'With practical information, real world data and case studies, David's book is a valuable contribution to the growing body of knowledge about green building, and will help the global property and construction industry's transition to a more sustainable future.'

ROMILLY MADEW

Chief Executive of Green Building Council of Australia

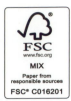

© David H. Clark / Cundall Johnston & Partners LLP, 2013

Published by RIBA Publishing,
15 Bonhill Street, London EC2P 2EA

ISBN 978 1 85946 447 2

Stock code 775531

British Library Cataloguing in Publications Data
A catalogue record for this book is available from the British Library.

Designed and typeset by: Alex Lazarou
Printed and bound by: W&G Baird Ltd, Antrim

RIBA Publishing is part of RIBA Enterprises Ltd.
www.ribaenterprises.com

Contents

Foreword

Cities are powerful engines of productivity. But they face enormous challenges from shifting demographics, the demand to reduce dependence on commodities, a changing climate, and the need to create an environment conducive to the improvement of human well-being.

Globally, there will be a continuing rural to urban shift of the population over the coming half-century. While the global population is in the process of stabilising, and is likely to level out at 9 billion by mid-century, the explosion of middle-class consumers, (those who spend between $10 and $100 a day) is unprecedented. At the turn-of-the-century there were around 1 billion middle class members of the global population. Now, just 13 years later, the number has doubled to 2 billion. That number is set to rise to about 5 billion by the year 2030. Most of these middle-class consumers will be urban dwellers.

Although this growth in the middle class is happening in the developing world, the impact is already being felt in the developed world. In a globalised economy we are all competing for the same resources, particularly for energy, water, food and minerals. Already, the basket of commodity prices which includes energy, food and minerals, is far higher than it has been over the past century. In order to meet this growing, new 21st-century challenge, there are two things we have to do. We must reduce the environmental footprint of our cities, and we must move to a circular economy in which commodities are recycled, remanufactured and returned to the marketplace. The era of wasteful disposal of valuable natural assets must end.

Buildings are a major part of the UK's carbon footprint. As such, they represent one of the most cost-effective opportunities for reducing CO_2 emissions, and also for reducing the country's dependence on imported energy sources. The current quality of our built environment leaves plenty of room for improvement. We must abandon the idea of 'energy consumption', 'materials and location', and 'transport' as separate issues. A holistic, systems analysis, approach leads to a more complex, but more useful, understanding of the challenges we face, and their potential solutions. Progress depends on clear thinking and ingenuity as well as access to sound data and information.

This book has a key role to play in the development of this important new approach to sustainable urban environments, fit for the future. Using clear, transparent data, it places in context the energy and CO_2 emissions associated with the construction and operation of buildings. But more than that, it challenges all those involved in the built environment – policy makers, planners, designers, builders, managers and occupants – to focus on the issues that make a difference. This book is an accessible, practical guide to reducing energy consumption and CO_2 emissions, providing a fresh approach but grounded in commercially available technologies.

Sir David King

Chair, Future Cities Catapult
Senior Science Adviser, UBS
Former Chief Scientific Adviser to the UK Government

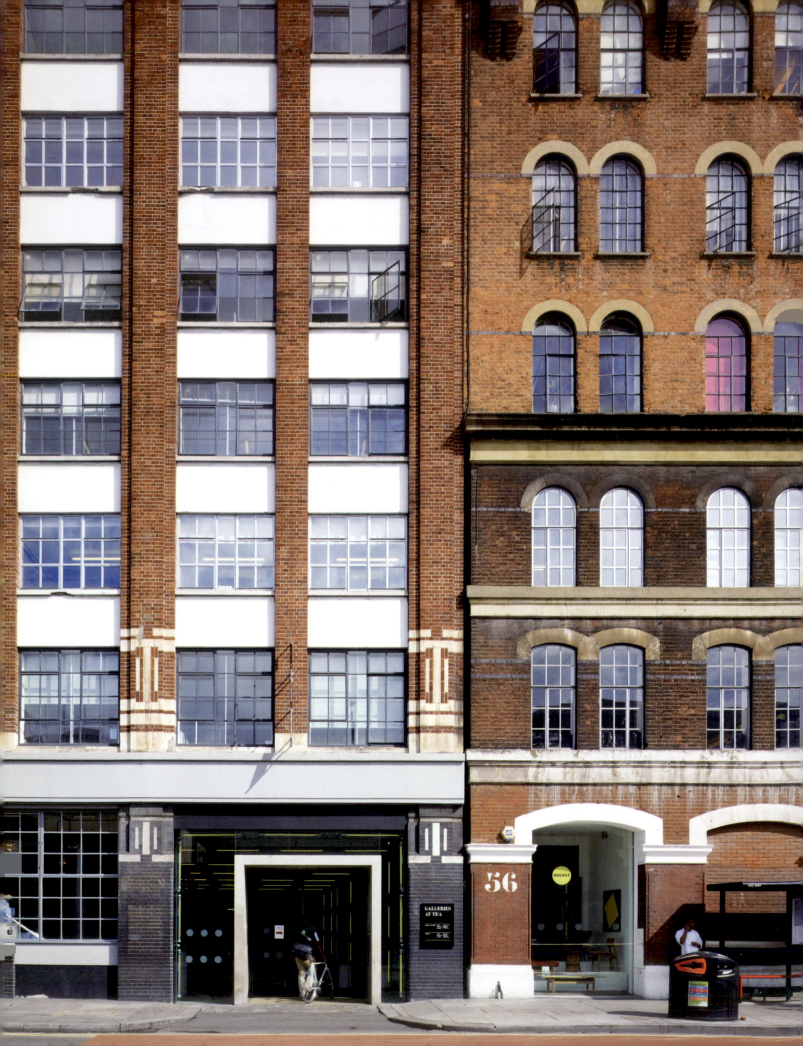

Introduction

People using buildings use energy, constructing and refurbishing buildings requires energy, and commuting to and from buildings consumes energy. Nearly all of this energy comes from the combustion of fossil fuels, which release greenhouse gases into the atmosphere.

The purpose of this book is to quantify the energy consumption and whole carbon footprint of buildings, primarily offices, and to provide practical guidance on how to reduce these. The footprint comprises:

- **operating** – the electricity, gas and other fuels used in a building for heating, cooling, ventilation, lighting, hot water, computers, servers and other equipment
- **embodied** – the energy consumed in manufacturing, delivering and installing the materials used to build, refurbish and fit-out a building, and their disposal at end of life
- **transport** – the energy used to get people to and from a building.

The footprint is quantified using kilograms of carbon dioxide equivalent $(kgCO_2e)$[1] which allows different forms of energy consumption – electrical, heat, embodied and motive (transport) – to be compared using a single metric. In the United Kingdom and many other countries, it provides a reasonable proxy to measure how efficiently energy is being used.[2]

ENERGY RESOURCES AND CLIMATE CHANGE

The global demand for fossil fuels continues to increase each year, while finding new reserves and extracting them cheaply and safely is becoming more difficult. Put simply, there is a finite supply of fossil fuel and we are using it up. Add global politics into the mix and it is inevitable that both energy prices and concerns over security of energy supply will increase. Buildings use 30 to 40% of global energy.[3] Reducing energy consumption and reliance on fossil fuels will therefore become more important in the property sector in the future, driven by a combination of building value, rising energy costs, profitability and legislation.

Then there is global warming and climate change. The overwhelming scientific consensus is that the increasing concentration of greenhouse gases in the atmosphere (mainly CO_2) is due to human activity and that this has raised, and will continue to raise, the average global surface temperature and change the world's climate.[4] Buildings contribute approximately one-third of global greenhouse gas emissions.

Whether you believe in the current theories on climate change or not is probably not particularly important. The legislation, financial drivers and solutions to reducing energy consumption and reliance on fossil fuels in buildings are mostly the same as those for reducing greenhouse gas emissions anyway.

VIRTUAL REALITY AND ACTUAL CONSUMPTION

Legislation has been introduced so that, by 2020, the design and construction of new buildings will be 'zero carbon' in the UK and 'nearly zero energy' in the European Union (EU). The definitions of these terms are still vague but the intention is clear – buildings in the future must be designed to be far more energy efficient and to utilise low-carbon energy sources.

While the focus on low energy/low carbon design is welcome, there is little consistent data published on how much energy buildings actually consume during operation. Do they work as intended? Do they provide good examples of how to reduce energy consumption in practice? Are the occupants engaged in saving energy? There is usually a large gap between design energy ratings and case studies, and actual energy consumption. The property sector needs to move away from good intentions and start to demonstrably reduce energy use and greenhouse gas emissions.

And what about the typical buildings that have been around for 10 years or more and will still be standing in 2050 – how much energy do they consume? Is it possible to halve the energy consumption of existing buildings? Should we knock them down and build newer, more efficient buildings? How much will the property sector have to rely on the decarbonisation of electricity grids to achieve significant greenhouse gas reductions by 2050?

Until real energy data is published consistently, and by everyone, the property industry will be unable to demonstrate that any progress is being made. The mandatory public reporting and display of real energy consumption in commercial buildings is long overdue in most countries.

EMBODIED CARBON

The calculation of embodied carbon for construction, refurbishment and fit-out (the energy used to make and transport materials) is unregulated and open to interpretation. If the property sector struggles to consistently report and benchmark something as comparatively simple as annual energy consumption, then how will it cope with the complexity of embodied carbon over the lifespan of the building?

There are already many methodologies, of varying complexity, to estimate embodied carbon, but how accurate does the estimation need to be to inform design decisions? How much of the whole carbon footprint does embodied carbon account for over the expected life of a building anyway? Will making detailed and expensive embodied carbon assessments radically change how buildings are constructed (timber and straw bale skyscrapers anyone?) or should the focus be on implementing practical ways to reduce embodied carbon by targeting the biggest contributors?

Finally, if a new building is constructed to meet future zero carbon design standards in the UK, this does not mean that embodied carbon will then account for 100% of its carbon footprint. Proponents of zero carbon buildings usually ignore two things – real buildings use far more energy than legislative design software predicts, and people also have to travel to get to work.

LOCATION, LOCATION, LOCATION

The location of a building is usually overlooked when considering energy resource consumption and greenhouse gas emissions. Many new buildings in city centres are large, sealed, high-rise glass boxes which rely heavily on air conditioning and artificial lighting to provide acceptable conditions for the occupants. They often have excessive energy consumption and limited opportunities for on-site renewable energy generation. However, a large proportion of their occupants travel to work by public transport.

Compare these with exemplar green buildings located away from city centres which have the flexibility and space to incorporate natural ventilation, daylighting, on-site renewable energy and so on. They might be low carbon, but, if most people have to drive there, should the greenhouse gas emissions from their cars be ignored when comparing their green credentials to city centre buildings?

RATING TOOLS DON'T TELL THE WHOLE STORY

There are numerous rating tools to benchmark energy performance and the environmental credentials of buildings, but none quantify the whole carbon footprint using a single, transparent metric. Most of the tools are based on computer modelling of energy and not the actual performance of real buildings occupied by real people. To illustrate this issue, consider which of these office buildings in the UK has the lowest whole carbon footprint – and how would you know?

A   A new timber-framed naturally ventilated building in a rural location with 50% on-site renewable energy systems and an A-rated Energy Performance Certificate (EPC).

B   A new steel and concrete BREEAM Excellent building with limited car parking in the centre of Birmingham.

C   A refurbished 1960s building in the centre of London with a D-rated Display Energy Certificate (DEC).

Note: for other countries, substitute EPC (modelled energy), DEC (metered energy) and BREEAM (environmental design rating) with equivalent rating tools such as Energy Star, NABERS, LEED and Green Star.

Building A sounds impressive, but an EPC rating is based on a computer simulation of how some parts of the building might perform in a perfect world. It does not, and was never intended to, predict the total energy consumption of the building. The rural location suggests there may be a reliance on cars for commuting.

Building B has a BREEAM Excellent rating, but energy is only one part of the rating (typically around one-fifth of the total available score). The energy score is based on the same modelling as that used to calculate an EPC, plus extra points for various initiatives, such as metering. It is a design rating and not based on actual energy consumption.

So, only for Building C is there any indication of how much energy is actually being used, because DECs are based on annual metered energy consumption. There is almost no correlation between EPC and DEC ratings for office buildings as they are based on different methodologies and benchmarks. Even assuming that Building A has an A-rated DEC (close to zero operating CO_2), would it have a lower whole carbon footprint than Building C when embodied carbon and greenhouse gas emissions due to commuting are taken into account?

There is currently no internationally agreed methodology for measuring the whole carbon footprint of buildings. Without this, how can we be sure that we are making the right decisions when planning how the built environment (as well as individual buildings) should respond to the energy and climate change challenges?

WHY WAS THIS BOOK WRITTEN?

The author's search for answers to the issues raised above led to the question: What is the contribution of operating, embodied and transport energy to the whole carbon footprint of buildings? Part 1 of this book puts these three components into perspective for offices buildings and then proposes a simple, transparent methodology to assess the whole carbon footprint.

However, quantifying the footprint is meaningless if it does not then lead to action to reduce energy consumption and greenhouse gas emissions. Part 2 of the book provides guidance to assist developers, building owners, occupiers, designers, planners and policy makers in reducing the whole carbon footprint of buildings.

LIMITATIONS

This book is primarily for office buildings but most of the principles can be applied, or can be adapted, to other building types. The focus on energy consumption and greenhouse gas emissions does not imply that other environmental and social issues are not important. Many of these are touched upon at various points in the book, including indoor environment, waste, natural resource consumption, preservation of ecology and water conservation, where they overlap with energy and carbon considerations. It was simply beyond the scope of the book to cover them in detail.[5]

The author currently resides in the UK and previously spent 14 years working in Australia, and the book reflects this experience. While the book has a strong UK bias in terms of legislation, data and climate, the principles can be applied to buildings in most countries. This isn't much of a stretch – new office buildings tend to look the same the world over anyway.

How the book is structured

Part 1 – What colour?

Part 1 describes how to calculate and benchmark the whole carbon footprint of buildings.

Chapter 1 introduces global issues with energy and climate change, examines the contribution that buildings make and establishes why $kgCO_2e$ is adopted as the unit of measurement for the carbon footprint in this book.

Chapter 2 evaluates the actual (not design) energy performance of office buildings and proposes that benchmarks should be based on occupied area and occupancy, with separate ratings for landlords and tenants.

Chapter 3 delves into the dark art of calculating embodied carbon, provides typical values that can be used for quick estimates and compares this with operating carbon over a 60-year lifespan.

Chapter 4 discusses how location influences the way that people choose to travel to a building, and compares commuting CO_2e emissions for a typical city centre building with out-of-town locations.

Chapter 5 combines the operating, embodied and transport CO_2e emissions into a whole carbon footprint, with indicative benchmarks. A simple benchmarking tool can be downloaded from **www.wholecarbonfootprint.com**.

Part 2 – Changing colour

Part 2 of the book presents approaches and solutions to reducing the energy consumption and carbon footprint of buildings.

Chapter 6 outlines ten steps to low energy consumption, including addressing our expectations of buildings, how they are managed and maintained, and the design/selection of building fabric, heating, cooling, ventilation, lighting and equipment.

Chapter 7 assesses the contribution that renewable energy systems can realistically make to reduce CO_2e emissions in individual buildings and asks 'Is it possible to make an urban building zero carbon using on-site renewables?'

Chapter 8 describes a pragmatic approach to reducing the embodied carbon of buildings and fit-outs, providing guidance on how to specify low-carbon materials and products and how to reduce CO_2e emissions associated with construction activities.

Chapter 9 discusses how building owners and tenants can encourage the use of greener modes of transport for commuting and business travel.

Chapter 10 outlines the potential ingredients to incorporate into a business case for investment in low-carbon buildings and refurbishments, including cost of occupancy and occupants, financial incentives and building value.

Appendices

The appendices to the book are published in electronic format only and can be downloaded from **www.whatcolourisyourbuilding.com**. They provide calculations, background information and further detail on the topics covered in the ten chapters of this book.

A   Energy, CO_2 and climate change
B CO_2e emission factors
C   Energy consumption data
D   Operating energy rating methodology
E   Embodied carbon data
F   Transport carbon data
G   Whole carbon footprint benchmarking
H   Reducing operating carbon
I   Renewable energy data
J   Materials data
K   Travel planning
L   Financial incentives
M   Building X and Hotel Y

Information papers

Various information papers are referenced in the book and appendices. They contain technical details, additional data and/or research on specific topics and can be downloaded from the website **www.wholecarbonfootprint.com**. They do not form part of the book and may be updated over time.

1. Security of energy supply
2. Adapting buildings to climate change
3. Fuel mix in grid electricity
4. CO_2e emissions from biomass & biofuels
5. Emission factors for black carbon
6. CO_2e emissions due to office waste
7. Analysis of display energy certificates 2008–10
8. US office energy data
9. Design energy rating data
10. Area and age of UK office stock
11. Comparison of building energy benchmark to total UK energy
12. Embodied carbon case studies for office buildings
13. Embodied carbon standards
14. Land use efficiency – city centre versus rural
15. Whole carbon footprint in rating tools
16. Heating degree days
17. Thermal comfort standards
18. Types of blinds for offices
19. Facade modelling – daylight and thermal performance
20. Ventilation rates in offices – mechanical and natural
21. Overview of HVAC systems in office buildings
22. Chiller energy efficiency
23. Solar hot water types & efficiencies
24. Photoltaic panel types and efficiencies
25. Biomass and biofuel sources
26. Wind speed data
27. Wind turbine performance
28. CHP types and efficiencies
29. CHP calculations
30. UK Government incentives for renewable energy
31. Embodied carbon of steel versus concrete buildings
32. Corporate attitudes to sustainability
33. Productivity in office buildings
34. The green premium – is it real?
35. The rising cost of energy and carbon
36. Useful daylight index

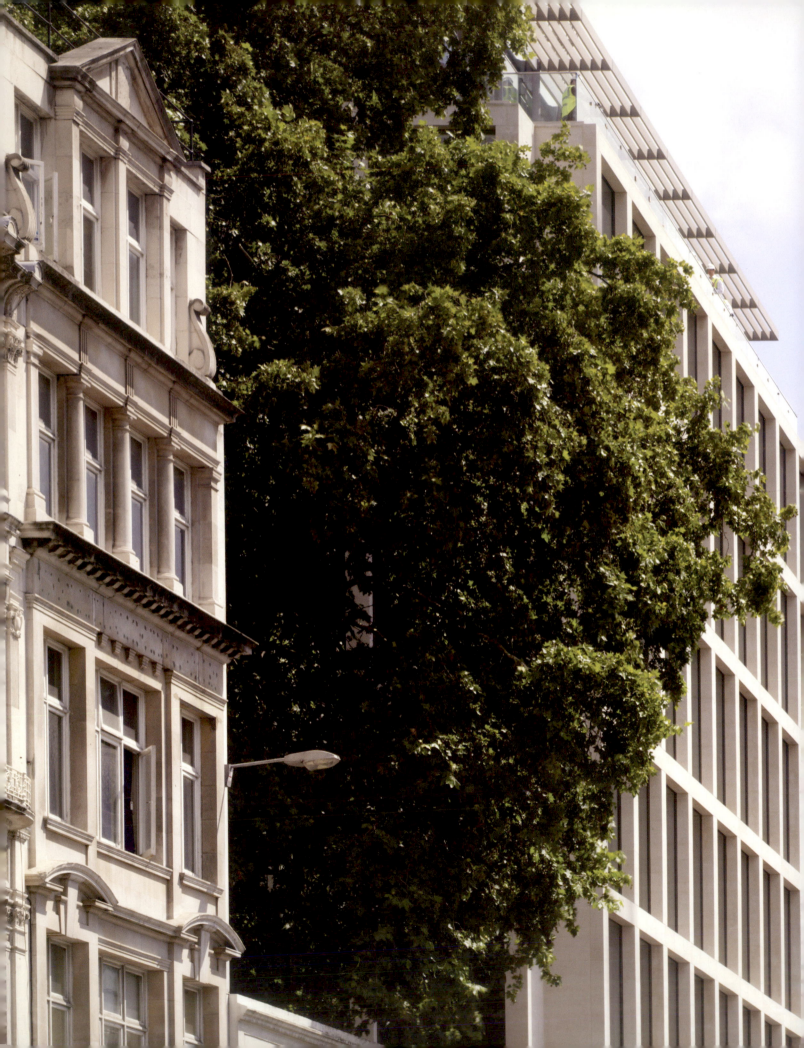

Part 1

WHAT COLOUR?
Measuring energy and carbon in buildings

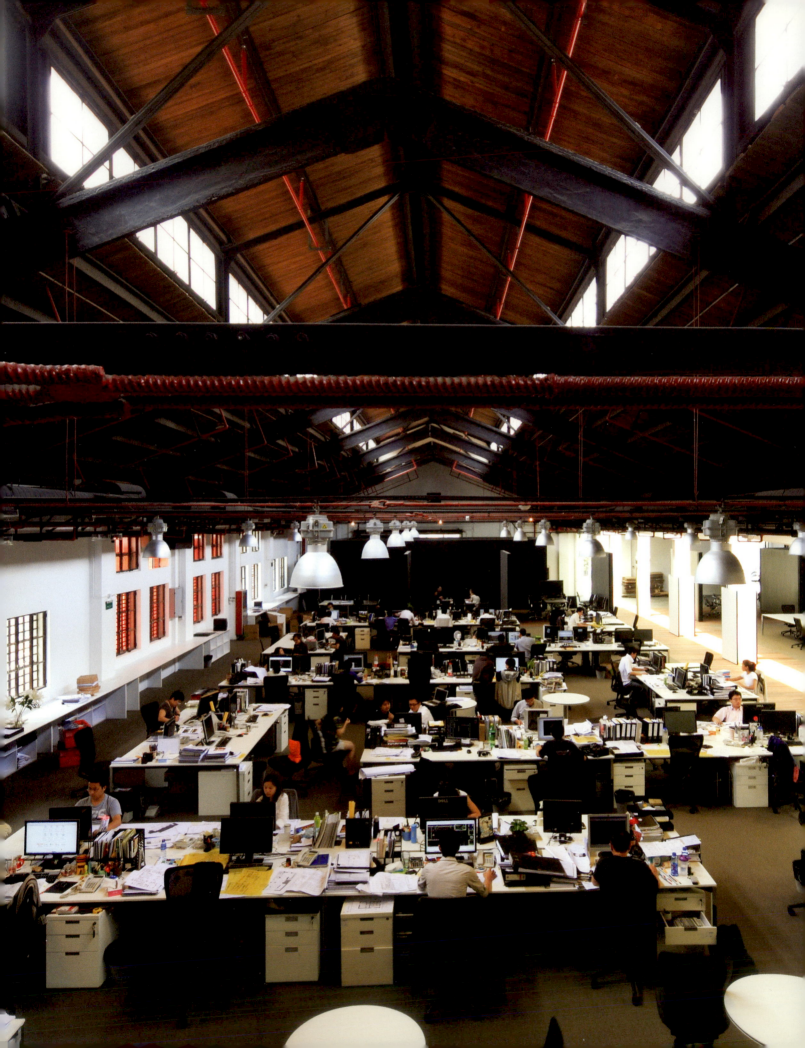

Chapter One

Energy and carbon in buildings

The world has achieved brilliance without wisdom, power without conscience. Ours is a world of nuclear giants and ethical infants … If we continue to develop our technology without wisdom or prudence, our servant may prove to be our executioner.

General Omar Bradley
An Armistice Day Address (10 November 1948), published in
The Collected Writings Of General Omar N. Bradley, Volume 1 (1967)

1.1 THE GLOBAL ENERGY CHALLENGE

Rising energy consumption

Global energy consumption is a function of three factors: the number of consumers (people), their demand for services (expectations) and the efficiency with which the services are provided (efficiency). A pseudo equation for this, which applies at building, city and global scales, is:

$$\text{Energy consumption} = \frac{\text{no. of people} \times \text{expectations}}{\text{efficiency}}$$

The global population is predicted to increase by 25% over the next two decades, from 6.9 billion in 2010 to 8.6 billion in 2035, with nearly all this growth occurring in the urban areas of developing countries.[1] More people means more energy consumption. At the same time, people's incomes in developing countries are rising, leading to further demands for energy as their expectations increase. The high-income Western lifestyle consumes a lot of energy (cars, large TVs, numerous gadgets, big fridges, air conditioning, flights overseas, comfortable houses and so on) and people in other countries want some of this too.

In high-income countries the average energy consumption in 2010 was 159 kWh per person per day (kWh/p/d), in lower middle income countries it was only 21 kWh/p/d and the world average was 59 kWh/p/d.[2] In just 10 years since 2000, China's consumption almost doubled from 30 kWh/p/d to 58 kWh/p/d. This is still half the per capita energy consumption of the UK and less than one-quarter of the USA's. What will happen when billions more people double their energy consumption?

The final factor is efficiency. History suggests, somewhat counter-intuitively, that as we improve energy efficiency, rather than reducing energy consumption it often goes up. For example, as cars became more efficient we could afford to drive further, and efficient gas central heating allows all rooms to be heated to higher temperatures for longer periods rather than using a single gas fire to heat one or two rooms. This effect is known as the Jevons Paradox.[3] To counter it, as efficiency increases then the cost of energy also needs to rise so that the net cost to the consumer of using the product or service remains the same while energy consumption reduces. Will this be politically palatable?

Reducing the global demand for energy is therefore a huge challenge. Between 2010 and 2035 it is predicted that energy consumption will increase by one-third, and that is assuming governments actually implement their current energy and climate policies (rather than just talking about them).[4] Buildings account for around 40% of global energy consumption[5] and will therefore have to be a major part of the energy solution.

Reliance on fossil fuels

Coal accounted for nearly half of the 25% increase in global energy use between 2000 and 2010, with the bulk of the growth coming from the power sector in emerging economies. Over 80% of the demand for energy in 2010 was supplied from fossil fuels and current predictions suggest that it will still account for 75% in 2035.[6]

Fossil fuels are a finite resource – it's just that no one can agree on how much there is remaining, how long it will last and what the cost to consumers will be. While oil supply diversity is diminishing, new technologies are opening up previously unviable reserves, such as shale gas. The Deepwater Horizon oil spill disaster in the Gulf of Mexico in 2010 and the groundwater pollution concerns raised by the fracking techniques used to extract shale gas are reminders that extracting fossil fuels is not without economic, social and environmental risk.[7]

The significant changes in lifestyle and economic prosperity that have occurred in the 250 years since the Industrial Revolution, have been built on fossil fuels. It is going to be very difficult to wean the world off this resource. While fossil fuels will not run out in the next 50 years, new reserves of fossil fuels that are cheap and easy to extract are becoming harder to find. This, combined with increasing consumption, will lead to more competition for energy, which will result in higher energy prices.

ENERGY AND OTHER ENVIRONMENTAL ISSUES

In addition to greenhouse gas emissions, other impacts associated with the use of energy include air pollution, water pollution, loss of biodiversity and habitat, visual or noise pollution and deforestation. These issues are not limited to fossil fuels: wind turbines are visually obtrusive, biomass releases particulates, plantations for biofuel can cause deforestation or replacement of food crops, hydro schemes can lead to major relocation of people and flooding of habitat, and nuclear power has issues related to fallout and the safe storage of radioactive waste for thousands of years. Most energy sources have localised environmental or social impacts – the problem with fossil fuels is that their climate change impact is also global.

Security of supply

Securing a reliable and diverse energy supply in the future is now a major concern in many countries. The European Union's Climate and Energy Policy states that the EU needs more secure energy sources, and to be less dependent on imports of foreign oil and gas, so as to make it less vulnerable to volatile energy prices and uncertain supply chains.[8] The EU currently imports over half of its primary energy requirements and is wary of an overreliance on Russia to supply natural gas.[9] Between 2002 and 2009, the renewable sector grew by over 50% and currently accounts for around one-fifth of the EU's primary energy production, with the majority from biomass and waste.

The increased use of air conditioning, heat pumps, computers and, more recently, electric vehicles is increasing the demand for electricity. To provide a reliable supply of electricity requires significant investment in power stations and distribution infrastructure, but even with this, unexpected events can lead to power shortages. Should we be designing buildings that require a constant supply of grid electricity to remain habitable?

CO_2 and global warming

When fuel is converted into energy to power buildings, industry and transportation it releases greenhouse gases (GHG). The amount of GHG emitted depends on the type of fuel used.[10]

GHG emissions = energy x carbon content of fuel

The radiative forcing of the climate system, which causes global warming, is dominated by increasing atmospheric concentrations of greenhouse gases, primarily due to carbon dioxide (CO_2) from human activities. While the scientific understanding of this is well-established, the global warming and cooling effects due to other factors, including black carbon, cloud albedo (reflectivity) and aerosols is less well understood. There are then further challenges in determining how the rising global temperatures will actually change local climates. Figure 1.1 summarises the main mechanisms in climate change science.[11]

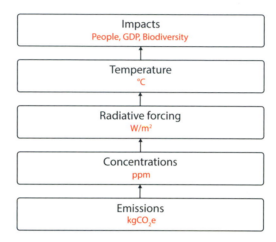

Fig 1.1 **The five key components in the science of climate change**

Climate change science is complex and predicting the future is difficult, confusing and full of uncertainties. This opens the door to lots of different opinions, running the full spectrum from 'the end of the world is nigh', to 'there's nothing to worry about; it's only natural'. According to the Intergovernmental Panel on Climate Change (IPCC), global warming is real, man-made and will have a serious impact on humans and the environment this century.

There is currently broad scientific and political consensus that global warming since 1750 (the start of the Industrial Revolution) must be kept below 2 °C to avert dangerous climate change. This requires greenhouse gas concentrations in the atmosphere to be limited to 450 parts per million (ppm). In 1750, they stood at 280 ppm and in 2010 had risen to 390 ppm, far in excess of the natural range of the last 650,000 years. To achieve the 450 ppm target, there is a general scientific agreement that worldwide emissions must stop rising by 2020, must be cut by at least half of their 1990 levels by 2050, and must continue to fall thereafter. In 2010, emissions were 49% higher than in 1990 and continue to rise each year.[12] In 2009, over 100 countries signed the Copenhagen Accord adopting the 2 °C target.[13] This will eventually lead to more stringent legislation and a higher cost on CO_2 emissions through the pricing of carbon.

Buildings are interlinked with global warming and climate policy in a number of ways:

- they contribute 30% of the world's CO_2 emissions[14]
- the cost of carbon will impact on running costs, the price of construction materials and the cost of travelling between buildings
- they need to adapt to changing climates in the future (potentially higher temperatures and more extreme weather events).

ADAPT AND SURVIVE

Whatever the reason, the climate is changing. Weather events are continually becoming more severe with records broken every year: the wettest summer for 100 years, the hottest year since records began, the highest number of hurricanes in a season, and so on. Insurance companies are acutely aware of this as they have to pick up the bills to repair the damage caused.[15] Adapting to the already unavoidable changes in climate over the next 50 to 100 years will affect both new and existing buildings.

Climate adaptation is a big issue and will trigger a fundamental shift in how design is approached, by moving from rules based on past experience to those based on future climate projections. Research on how best to achieve this without increasing energy consumption (Figure 1.2 shows a simplistic scenario) is still in its early days.[16]

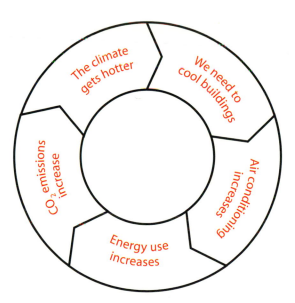

Fig 1.2 **A downward spiral? Climate adaptation could lead to increasing CO_2 emissions**

Different issues – same solutions?

To reduce greenhouse gas emissions due to buildings, manufacturing and transportation requires a reduction in energy consumption and an increase in alternative energy sources. These are the same solutions as those required to resolve our energy resource and security of supply issues. So, it doesn't really matter if you are a climate-change sceptic or not, the need to act and the issues to address are similar.

Unfortunately, the world's politicians (and the majority of voters) can't currently agree whose problem it is, how to fix it, how much it will cost, when to start, or who will pay. This lack of urgency, despite the overwhelming scientific consensus on the need to act decisively now, could be because the main consequences will not impact on communities and economies immediately. Instead, they will occur sometime in the future (after the next couple of election cycles) and mainly affect someone else (our descendants who currently can't vote, or people in a different country).

The political reality is that legislation to make reductions will gradually become more stringent in some countries, but the vital radical transformation in global energy supply and consumption is unlikely to occur within the timeframes required to limit climate change to 2 °C. As Admiral Hyman Rickover observed in 1957, 'High energy consumption has always been a prerequisite of political power'.[17]

Despite this doom and gloom, it is not too late for individuals and companies to show leadership, make a difference and gain commercial advantage. The property sector does not have to wait for government legislation to make significant energy savings and greenhouse gas reductions – there is already plenty of low hanging fruit available. Part 2 of this book provides guidance on where it is and how to take it.

1.2 BUILDINGS ARE PART OF THE SOLUTION

'Buildings use approximately 40% of global energy consumption and release 30% of global CO_2 emissions.' This should really say 'People using buildings use …' Occupants have a major influence on how buildings perform – it's not just about technology.

Over the next 20 years, energy consumption in buildings globally is predicted to double.[18] Limiting this increase will therefore be essential if any international climate change strategy is to be successful. While a globally enforced agreement may be some time in coming, many countries have acknowledged the need for action and have begun to introduce legislation targeting various sectors, including buildings.

Energy legislation in the property sector has tended to focus on the design and construction of new buildings, through building regulations and the planning approval process. However, since almost three-quarters of the non-domestic buildings standing in 2010 will still be standing in 2050 (representing 60% of the building stock), there is an increasing recognition of the need to significantly reduce the energy consumption of existing buildings too.[19]

It is not only legislation that is driving energy and CO_2 reduction in buildings. The rapid growth in Green Building Councils around the world, from two in 2002 to over 80 in 2012,[20] and the voluntary use of environmental rating tools such as BREEAM, LEED and Green Star, shows that many players in the property industry are acknowledging that there is a need to act.

In order for buildings to become part of the solution to reducing global energy consumption and GHG emissions, a clear understanding of their contribution to the problem is needed:

- How do buildings use energy and influence energy use?
- How can this be measured?

1.3 WHERE DO GHG EMISSIONS OCCUR IN BUILDINGS?

The terms 'operating carbon', 'embodied carbon' and 'transport carbon' are used throughout this book. In this context, carbon is shorthand for 'carbon dioxide equivalent (CO_2e) emissions', which will be discussed shortly. Figure 1.3 (overleaf) provides a simplified picture of where these emissions occur during the construction and operation of a typical building.

Operating energy and CO_2e emissions

Buildings use two forms of energy – electricity and heat. Electricity is typically sourced from the national electricity grid. Heat is usually generated in the building using one, or a combination, of the following: electricity, gas (natural or LPG), biomass, biofuel, diesel or oil, although in some locations district heating networks are used. The consumption of energy releases GHG emissions, either at the building (e.g. gas boiler) or at the power stations supplying the building.

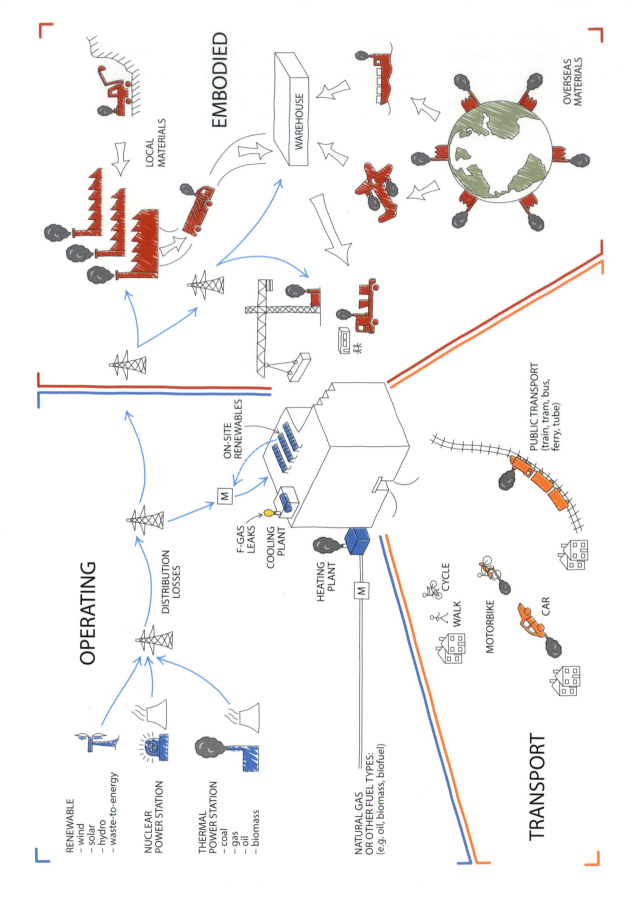

Fig 1.3 GHG emissions associated with the construction and occupancy of buildings

Measuring energy consumption

The unit for energy consumption that is used in this book is a kilowatt-hour (kWh). To put a kWh into perspective, a 40 watt lamp turned on for 24 hours consumes approximately 1 kWh. To convert kWh to other units, such as megajoules (MJ), British thermal units (Btu) and tonnes of oil equivalent (toe), refer to Appendix A.

Measuring GHG emissions

The unit for GHG emissions used in this book is kilograms of carbon dioxide equivalent ($kgCO_2e$). 1 $kgCO_2e$ is equivalent to the global warming potential of 1 kilogram of carbon dioxide over a 100-year period.[21] Calculating the annual CO_2e emissions due to energy consumption is relatively straightforward:

- Work out the total energy consumption for each energy source by reading the electricity and gas meters (or, for other fuels, measure the volume/weight consumed).
- Multiply these totals by the appropriate CO_2e emission factor (the $kgCO_2e$ per unit of energy consumed).

Unfortunately, there are many different published emission factors and these will give different results. The main variances are for:

- **grid electricity** – this varies by country, by year (due to the fuel mix used for power generation) and by calculation methodology
- **scope of emissions** – do the factors include the energy required to produce and deliver the energy to the consumer as well as the emissions due to combustion?

Converting energy consumption into CO_2e emissions

The emission factors used to convert kWh into $kgCO_2e$ for different energy sources and countries are discussed in detail in Appendix B. The key to benchmarking is to use consistent metrics so, in this book, the UK emission factors shown in Table 1.1 (overleaf) have been used. These are similar to average emission factors globally.[22] The reasons for using CO_2e to benchmark energy instead of using 'primary energy' are discussed at the end of this chapter.

Fuel	kgCO$_2$e/kWh
Grid electricity	**0.60**
Natural gas	**0.20**
Heating oil (kerosene)	0.31
Diesel	0.32
Petrol	0.30
LPG	0.26

Table 1.1 CO$_2$e emission factors used in this book

The CO$_2$e emission factors include the direct emissions when the fuels are combusted plus the emissions due to extraction, processing, manufacture, storage and delivery of fuels (the 'embodied energy'). The grid electricity factor also includes distribution losses of around 7.5%, due to average losses in the infrastructure between the power station and the end user.

These embodied emissions are often excluded from the emission factors used to benchmark energy consumption in buildings. Since this book is about the whole carbon footprint of buildings, including the embodied carbon of the building construction, it is appropriate that the embodied carbon used to produce the fuels used in buildings is also considered.

The emission factors for biomass and biofuels are more complex and depend on where the fuel is sourced, how much energy is used to process and transport the fuels and the assumptions made regarding reabsorption of the CO$_2$ emissions released during combustion by the trees and crops subsequently planted to replace the original fuel source. They may be renewable energy but they are not zero carbon, and indeed some biofuels have higher net CO$_2$e emissions than petrol. Appendix B provides further discussion and CO$_2$e emission factors for different types of biomass and biofuels.

The energy consumption and CO$_2$e emissions in office buildings are described in Chapter 2. Methods of reducing energy consumption and the use of renewable/low-carbon energy generation are discussed in Chapters 6 and 7 respectively.

Embodied energy and CO₂e emissions

This is a complex subject because of the large supply chain involved in the construction, fit-out, maintenance, refurbishment and eventual demolition of buildings. Every material or product used in a building has a carbon footprint due to the greenhouse gas emissions associated with material excavation, processing, manufacture, assembly, storage, transportation, installation, maintenance and its eventual disposal at end of life. Goods are sourced from all over the world and the emissions will vary for almost identical materials/products due to:

- the energy efficiency of the manufacturing process
- the carbon intensity of the electricity grid in the country of manufacture
- the distance the goods have to travel
- the mode of transportation.

Importing goods from overseas may reduce emissions in the purchasing country but the emissions due to manufacture haven't disappeared – greenhouse gases don't stop at national borders. According to the Carbon Trust, approximately 25% of all CO_2 emissions from human activities flow from one country to another in commodities and products.[23] Major developed economies are typically net importers of embodied carbon emissions, effectively outsourcing some of their emissions to developing countries. For example, in the UK, while production of CO_2 reduced by around 20% between 1990 and 2008, the UK's contribution towards global warming increased by 10% because the cuts in local emissions were outweighed by importing

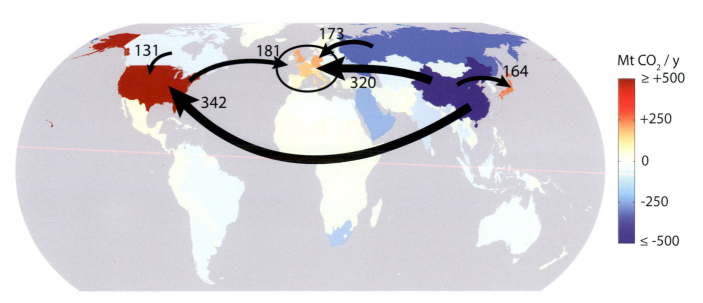

Fig 1.4 Carbon in trade (2004) – emissions embodied in products (source: Davis et al.)

more goods from overseas.[24] The UK may be meeting its own carbon budgets, but is it at the expense of the global carbon budget?

Figure 1.4 shows the carbon emissions embedded in products traded globally in 2004.[25] The arrows depict the largest interregional flows of emissions ($MtCO_2$/year) from net exporting countries to net importing countries; the threshold for arrows is 150 $MtCO_2$/year. Complaining about China's increasing GHG emissions, while buying lots of products from China could be considered to be hypocritical.

The embodied carbon of office buildings is described in Chapter 3 and the use of low-carbon materials to reduce this is discussed in Chapter 8.

Transport energy and CO_2e emissions

There are three main reasons to travel to and from buildings: to get to work, to visit (including business travel) and to deliver goods or services. The location of a building affects the travel distance of all three, but as visitors and goods deliveries are highly dependent on the type of businesses occupying a building, then it is not really feasible to include them in transport benchmarking of office buildings. Business travel, which can also include flying, can be readily incorporated into a company's carbon footprint and Corporate Social Reporting (CSR).[26]

From travel surveys it is possible to establish broad trends for commuting travel distances and modes of transport based on location, and consequently the annual average CO_2e emissions per person can be estimated. Buildings in city centres with good public transport and limited car parking spaces have fewer people driving to work compared to buildings out in the suburbs or edge-of-town business parks. The emission factors for different modes of transport, including cars, motorbikes, trains and buses, are given in Appendix B.

The CO_2e emissions due to commuting to office buildings are estimated in Chapter 4 and green travel opportunities are discussed in Chapter 9.

OTHER GLOBAL WARMING INFLUENCES DUE TO BUILDINGS

While global warming is dominated by the concentration of CO_2 in the atmosphere, buildings can contribute to warming in other ways:

- **Black carbon** – particulates (soot) from the incomplete combustion of fossil fuels and biomass contribute to global warming in two ways: in the atmosphere they add to the greenhouse effect, while on the ground they reduce the reflectivity of snow and ice. Black carbon's contribution to global warming is estimated to be approximately 10%, although recent research suggests it could be much higher.
- **F-gases** – these are potent greenhouse gases and include refrigerants leaking from air conditioning systems, heat pumps and fridges. For a typical air conditioned office building this might account for up to 2% of operating carbon emissions.
- **Methane from waste** – organic waste from office consumables going to landfill contributes to the release of methane. Some of this may be captured and used to produce energy.
- **Deforestation** – for buildings this typically relates to the reduction in CO_2 absorbing capacity of native forest due to unsustainable clear felling for construction timber or growing biofuel crops.

These factors are not included in the carbon footprint methodology described in this book because, compared to the main greenhouse gas emissions due to operating, embodied and transport energy, they are less straightforward to quantify. Emission factors for the first three, and how their contribution can be included in a building's carbon footprint if required, are described in Appendix B. Figure 1.5 shows the potential additional CO_2e emissions compared to operating energy in a typical UK office building.

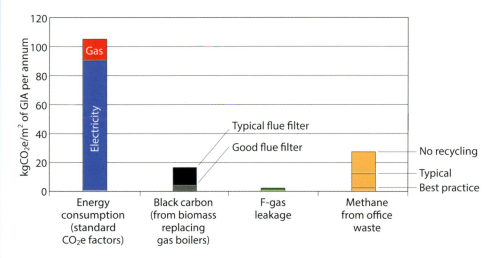

Fig 1.5 Potential CO_2e emissions due to other factors

1.4 MEASURING ENERGY AND GREENHOUSE GAS EMISSIONS

To make comparisons between operating, embodied and transport energy requires a consistent unit. There are two contenders:

- primary energy (kWh)
- carbon dioxide equivalent ($kgCO_2e$).

Primary energy is the energy that exists in a naturally occurring form, such as coal, oil and natural gas, that has not been subjected to any conversion or transformation process, such as refined fuels and electricity generation. The conversion factors from energy consumed to primary energy and CO_2e emissions for natural gas and grid electricity are shown in Table 1.2. Also shown are typical domestic and commercial office energy tariffs in the UK in 2012.

	GHG Emissions (kgCO₂e/ kWh)	Primary energy[27] (kWh(PE)/kWh)			Typical tariffs[28] (p/kWh)	
		Passivhaus	SAP 2009	US Energy Star	Domestic	Office
Grid electricity	0.6	2.7	2.9	3.34	12.6p	10p
Natural gas	0.2	1.1	1.0	1.047	3.9p	3.5p
Ratio of electricity to gas	**3.0**	**2.5**	**2.9**	**3.2**	**3.2**	**2.9**

Table 1.2 Comparison of primary energy, CO_2e emissions and energy costs for gas and electricity consumed in buildings

In the UK there are not significant differences between the ratios of electricity and natural gas using CO_2e emission factors, primary energy factors and energy costs. As a proxy for energy resource consumption, CO_2e calculated using the emission factors in Table 1.1 seems pretty reasonable.

The use of $kgCO_2e$ as the unit of measurement therefore has been adopted in this book for the following reasons:

- many building energy rating tools use CO_2 as the metric[29]
- different forms of transport are typically compared by CO_2 emissions not primary energy
- reducing greenhouse gas emissions is a pressing environmental issue
- the ratio between the UK emission factors for gas and electricity is similar to that for primary energy.

In this book, the energy consumption of a building is sometimes expressed in $kgCO_2e$. While technically $kgCO_2e$ is not 'energy', it can become somewhat pedantic to keep referring to 'the greenhouse gas emissions due to operating energy consumption'.

1.5 SUMMARY

Global energy consumption is predicted to increase by 30% between 2010 and 2035, with fossil fuels providing 75% of the energy supply. This rising demand will create competition, leading to higher energy prices and security of supply issues because fossil fuels are not an unlimited resource. Many countries are seeking to limit their reliance on imported fossil fuels, and their exposure to energy cost increases, by both reducing energy consumption and investing in alternative energy sources, including renewables. This approach also conveniently reduces greenhouse gas emissions – the ultimate BOGOF.[29]

Buildings are responsible for 30% of the global greenhouse gas emissions and 40% of global energy consumption and so have a major role to play in government policies targeting reductions in both. Their influence is even greater when embodied and transport energy is considered.

Using CO_2e as a proxy for consumption of energy resources as well as a measure of greenhouse gas emissions, the whole energy and carbon footprint of a building is defined as the CO_2e emissions due to metered operating energy consumption, embodied energy in materials and transport energy used for commuting. The next four chapters aim to put these into perspective for office buildings, although the principles can be applied to other building types.

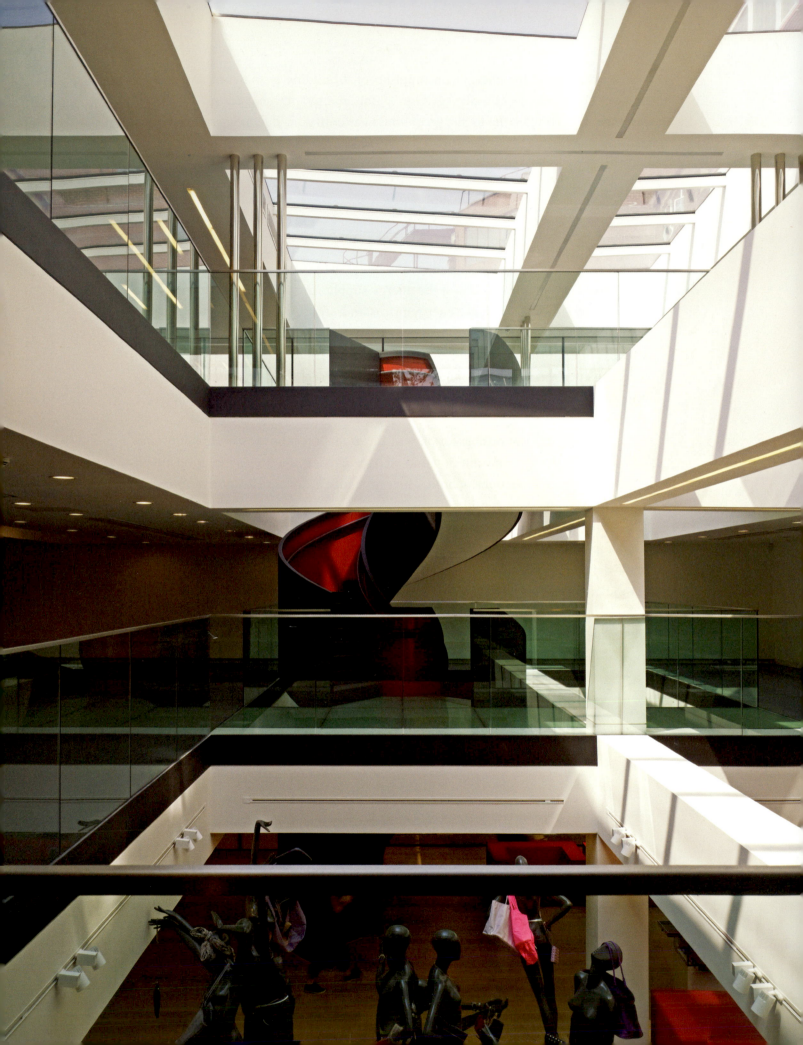

Chapter 2

How much energy do buildings use?

An ounce of performance is worth pounds of promises.
Mae West, American actress

2.1 METHODS OF MEASURING ENERGY CONSUMPTION

When buying a car, most of us will at some point consider the fuel economy, in either miles per gallon or litres per 100 km. We may then decide that it is not really that important in making our purchasing decision, but at least we'll have a reasonable idea of how often the tank will need to be filled, and how much this will cost each time. This is because fuel is a major cost in running a car and the fuel gauge is highly visible.

In most commercial office buildings, energy is a relatively small proportion of the total cost of occupancy, typically less than 10%, compared to rates, rent and landlord service charges.[1] Considering other costs, such as salaries, the cost of energy to most office-based businesses is hardly noticeable. It is perhaps, therefore, not surprising that occupants have limited understanding of how their building is performing – what the equivalent fuel economy is.

Determining the annual energy consumption of a building is relatively easy, provided you have access to the utility meters – simply take readings 12 months apart and calculate the difference. If a building has consumed 150,000 kWh of electricity and 75,000 kWh of gas in a year this gives a total of 225,000 kWh. This information is, however, of little use without something to compare or benchmark it against:

- What type of building is it?
- How big is it?
- How often is it used?
- How many occupants are there?
- Do the meters cover all the energy used?

- there is one person for every 15 m² of GIA[5]
- everyone works on a laptop with no extra screens
- the office is occupied between 8 a.m. and 6 p.m., Monday to Friday (50 hours per week)
- the office is required to be thermally comfortable all year round
- the occupants need fresh air, light, food, drink and sanitation
- the lifts are not used.

Energy in buildings is consumed by LEACHs, typically in the form of the following:

Lighting	*internal and external lights*
Equipment	*computers, printers, fridges, lifts, security systems, servers, etc.*
Air	*fans (supply and exhaust)*
Cooling	*chillers and pumps*
Heating	*space heating system, domestic hot water boiler and pumps*

Table 2.1 shows the breakdown of energy consumption based on the assumptions above.[6]

Item	Description	kWh/m² of GIA	kWh/person	% of total energy
Lights	Task lights and background ceiling lighting	8		16%
Equipment	Laptops, server, printers, kitchen	30		56%
Air **Cooling** **Heating**	High performance façade. Natural ventilation plus mechanical ventilation with heat recovery, heat pumps for heating/cooling to achieve Passivhaus Standards[7]	15		28%
	Total electrical energy consumption	**53**	**800**	
	Convert to primary energy (2.7 kWh$_{primary}$/kWh$_{final}$)	145	2,150	
		kgCO$_2$e/m² of GIA	kgCO$_2$e/ person	
	Convert to CO$_2$e emissions (0.6 kgCO$_2$e/kWh)	32	480	

Table 2.1 'Lowest energy office' consumption breakdown

This rough assessment, of what many would consider to be a cave with candles and abacuses, suggests that the lowest annual electrical energy consumption possible in 2013 in a fully occupied office is 53 kWh/m² or **32 kgCO$_2$e/m² of GIA**.

If the occupants want more powerful computers, two monitors, a few more cups of tea, 21 °C to 24 °C all year round, additional lighting, to use the lifts, to work longer hours or to cram more people into the office, then the energy consumption will increase.

If the office is only half occupied (one person per 30 m²) then the total energy consumption (and the energy by area) will reduce, but the energy per person will increase. If everyone had this amount of space we would need to build a lot more buildings. In many offices the server room can typically account for one-fifth of the building's electricity consumption.[8] Outsourcing some of the server functions to an external data centre will save energy in the office building, but simply transfers the energy consumption and associated CO_2e emissions elsewhere.

Figure 2.2 shows the net CO_2e emissions of the 'lowest energy office' for varying number of storeys, assuming that 50% of the roof area is covered with photovoltaic (PV) panels and the building is located in London.[9] Given that this is the 'lowest energy office' possible in 2013, the building is only zero carbon if it is single storey! The use of on-site renewables to provide energy and reduce CO_2e emissions in offices is covered in more detail in Chapter 7.

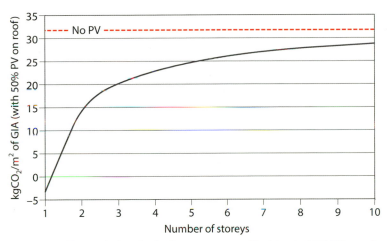

Fig 2.2 Net CO_2e emissions in the 'lowest energy office' due to 50% PV panels on the roof

So how does this theoretical 'lowest energy office' compare to real buildings?

CUNDALL'S MELBOURNE OFFICE

The author worked in the Melbourne office of Cundall, which occupied one floor of a five-storey building in the city centre, with a GIA of 195 m² and 12 staff (1 per 16 m²). In 2007, it had a total measured annual energy consumption of 13,100 kWh (all electricity) and was awarded a 5-star NABERS Tenancy rating. The landlord's lift and common area lighting was estimated to be an additional 3,100 kWh.

continued overleaf

continued

Converting the energy to CO_2e, using the emission factors in Chapter 1, gives:

$[16,200 \text{ kWh}/195\text{m}^2] \times EF = 83 \text{ kWh/m}^2 \times 0.60 = \textbf{50 kgCO}_2\textbf{e/m}^2$

$[16,200 \text{ kWh}/12] \times EF = 1,350 \text{ kWh/person} \times 0.60 = \textbf{810 kgCO}_2\textbf{e/person}$

The building had lots of daylight and thermal mass, openable windows, a reverse cycle air source heat pump (heating and cooling) and T8 fluorescent lighting with simple on/off switches. The building would fail nearly every energy efficiency requirement in modern building regulations (clear single glazing, electric immersion heater for hot water, large air gaps in the window frames, etc.) – but the occupants at the time were a hardy bunch. The ceiling lights were off most of the time (desk task lights were provided), ceiling fans helped with summer comfort,[10] jumpers were worn in winter and shorts in summer (when the external temperatures regularly exceeded 30 °C). The shower had a flow rate of just 4 litres per minute.

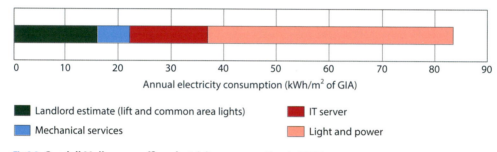

Annual electricity consumption (kWh/m² of GIA)

■ Landlord estimate (lift and common area lights)   ■ IT server

■ Mechanical services   ■ Light and power

Fig 2.3 **Cundall Melbourne office electricity consumption in 2007**

The air conditioning (heating and cooling) was on for a total of less than 30 hours in 2007. The heating, cooling, domestic hot water and toilet exhaust fans had a total sub-metered electricity consumption of just 6 kWh/m² despite none of them being energy efficient. The landlord's lights and lift (which were rarely used by Cundall) accounted for 20% of the total energy because the lights were left on 24/7.

This example illustrates that one of the biggest opportunities to save energy, even in inefficient buildings, is to make it easy to turn stuff off – something that many people forget when they are caught up in the complexity of designing modern buildings. If the office had been equipped with efficient lighting and computers (laptops), the landlord had turned the stair lights off at night and the air passing through the façade been more controlled, then it is possible that the 53 kWh/m² theoretical value in Table 2.1 could just have been achieved.

So the 'lowest possible energy' target is potentially achievable – but only in offices with some form of natural ventilation and occupants who embrace low energy principles (and wider thermal comfort bands). Unfortunately, it is not possible to fit a corporate headquarters into a small office and so this solution is not applicable for many city centre commercial office buildings.

2.3 ENERGY BENCHMARKS FOR OFFICE BUILDINGS

The Chartered Institution of Building Services Engineers (CIBSE) published energy benchmarks for 29 building categories in 2008 which were then incorporated into the UK Display Energy Certificate (DEC) scheme.[11] The office benchmark, adjusted to reflect the emission factors used in this book, is 81 $kgCO_2e/m^2$ of GIA.

DECs rate the energy performance of building occupants not landlords. This comprises their direct metered energy consumption plus a proportion of the landlord's energy consumption (heating, cooling, common areas, lifts, etc.), typically allocated based on the occupier's leased area compared to the total leasable area in the building. If a building has a single occupant then the DEC rating is effectively a whole building rating.

$$\text{DEC rating score} = \frac{\text{energy consumption} \times 100}{\text{energy benchmark}}$$

The DEC rating scale is shown in Figure 2.4 and is similar in appearance to energy labels used for appliances throughout the European Union. The energy benchmark gives a score of 100, which sits at the D/E boundary and not in the middle of the scale.

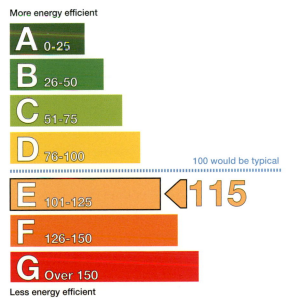

Fig 2.4 UK DEC rating for a building with 93 $kgCO_2e/m^2$

There are various adjustments that can be made to the energy consumption, such as excluding non-typical energy uses (known as allowable separables) and adjustments to the benchmark based on different uses in the building, hours of use and heating degree days.[12]

In 2003, the UK Government published the last version of the ECON 19 Energy Consumption Guide,[13] which gave a series of energy benchmarks for typical and good performance in four types of office building: natural ventilated (open plan and cellular buildings) and air conditioned (standard and prestige buildings).

Figure 2.5 shows the ECON 19 benchmarks and the theoretical 'lowest energy office' (from Table 2.1) superimposed on to the DEC rating scale.

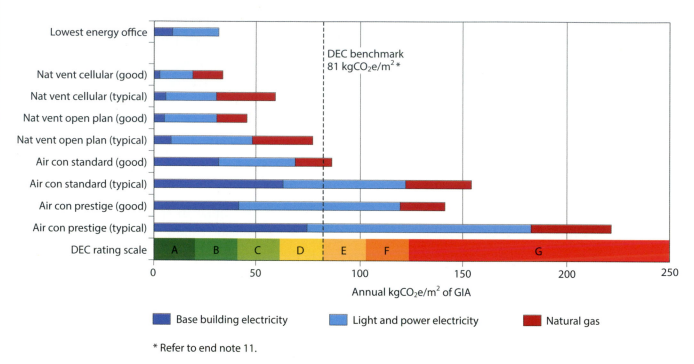

* Refer to end note 11.

Fig 2.5 **Lowest energy office and ECON 19 benchmarks superimposed on to the DEC rating scale**

All but the most efficient air conditioned buildings get a G rating, while naturally ventilated buildings can typically achieve a D rating or better. The lowest energy office has a B rating, and will only achieve an A rating if 50% of the roof area is covered with PV panels and the building is no higher than three storeys. The DEC rating scale is very onerous, which is probably due to it being primarily calibrated using public sector offices, the majority of which have natural ventilation.[14]

The voluntary uptake of DECs by the private sector has been low, which is primarily because, as suggested in Figure 2.5, most large prestige commercial offices will get a G rating. It is not a rating to proudly display in the foyer if your competitors aren't showing theirs.[15]

In comparison, the uptake of operating energy ratings by the commercial office sector in Australia (NABERS) and the USA (Energy Star) has been much more widespread.[16] The reasons include:

- Leases for government and large corporate tenants in Australia often include a requirement to deliver a minimum 4-star NABERS Energy base building rating.
- In 2011, it became mandatory to provide a NABERS rating certificate on the sale or lease of an office building over 2,000 m² in Australia. No minimum rating is set, but zero stars is not a great selling point.
- Tax and/or planning incentives are available in some states and cities in the USA for Energy Star rated buildings.[17]
- The ratings are more flattering than DECs – an 'Energy Star' sounds much better than a G rating.

Figure 2.6 shows an indicative comparison of the DEC, NABERS and Energy Star ratings for a whole building (landlord and tenant energy) in a similar climate. The red marks indicate the 'typical' (median) energy performance in each rating scale. A building classed as 'typical' using NABERS (2.5 stars) or Energy Star (50 points) would achieve a G rating in the UK. It is even possible for a building awarded Energy Star status in the USA to be equivalent to a G rating. This suggests that the Energy Star scale is probably not ambitious enough, rewarding mediocre performance, while the DEC rating scale does not have enough rating increments at the lower (D to G) end of the scale to differentiate (and therefore motivate) the occupants and landlords in air conditioned commercial buildings.

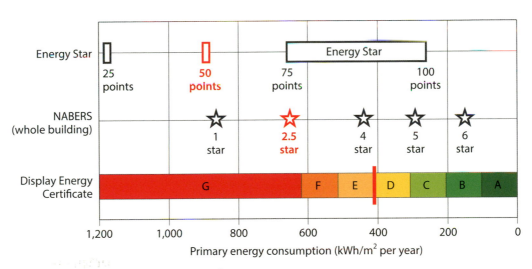

Note: the chart is in primary energy (kWh/m²) because the tools use different emissions factors to convert consumed energy to CO₂. The PE factors used were 3 for electricity and 1.1 for gas. The chart was based on an office with an electricity to gas energy consumption ratio (kWh) of 2 to 1, a gross to net floor area ratio of 1.25, an occupancy density of 1 per 12m² of NLA, 50 hours per week, and buildings located in London (DEC), Hobart (NABERS) and Seattle (Energy Star).

Fig 2.6 **Comparison of DEC, NABERS and Energy Star rating scales for a typical office building**

2.4 HOW DO TYPICAL OFFICE BUILDINGS PERFORM?

So far a lowest energy office and various benchmarks have been considered – but how much do typical office buildings actually consume? The energy performance published in books, articles and marketing material is usually based on energy modelling (for building regulations or design rating tools). Actual energy consumption data is difficult to obtain, and is often presented using different units and methodologies.

Table 2.2 lists a selection of operating energy data sources for office buildings. Figure 2.7 summarises this data after it has been converted, by the author, into the $kgCO_2e/m^2$ unit used in this book. Appendix C provides further details and commentary on this data.

Source	Year	Country	Total area (m^2)	Comments
Cundall offices	2010	UK	4,600	Data from energy audits of five Cundall UK offices
DEC database	2010	UK	9.6 million	Data is interpreted by the author from the Display Energy Certificate (DEC) database initially released under a Freedom of Information request
Better Buildings Partnership	2011	UK	> 1 million	Data provided to the author by the BBP for 138 London offices (with an average size of 9,200 m^2)
Energy Star Portfolio Manager	2012	USA	900 million	Data from US Environment Protection Agency (average energy star score was 62)
US Commercial Building Survey	2004	USA	Not known	Data from the US Energy Information Administration
New York City Energy Benchmarking	2011	USA	29.6 million	Data for 1,023 offices published to comply with Local Law 84 (897 of the buildings had Energy Star ratings)
Greenprint Index	2011	Various	28 million	Data for 1,628 commercial office properties in 46 countries

Table 2.2 Selection of sources of operating energy data in office buildings

The data in Figure 2.7 reveals a number of trends:

- naturally ventilated buildings tend to have lower energy consumption than air conditioned buildings
- the DEC ratings are primarily for public sector occupants, and this database shows lower energy consumption than the three commercial building databases
- the DEC benchmark of 81 $kgCO_2e/m^2$ does not represent average commercial office building performance.

The author proposes that 100 kgCO$_2$e/m^2 of GIA (using the emission factors in this book) be adopted as a typical benchmark when rating the performance of office buildings in the UK. This will also be used in Chapter 5 when considering the whole carbon footprint. It is worth noting that the majority of the buildings in Figure 2.7 were located in temperate zones. To establish appropriate benchmarks in other countries, the influence of climate on energy consumption and the energy sources used both need to be taken into consideration.

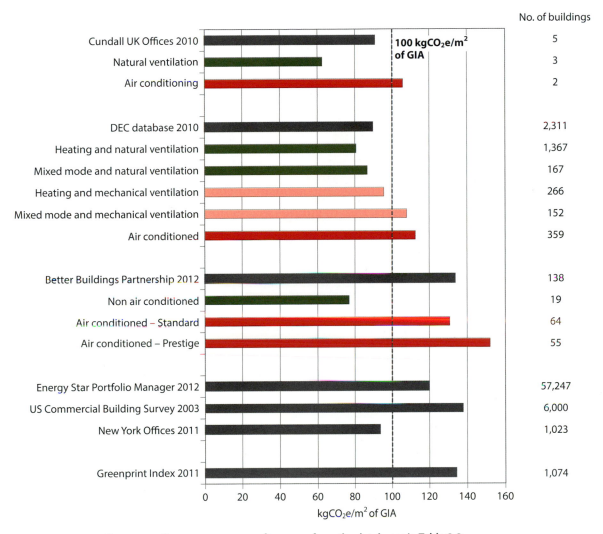

Fig 2.7 Summary of average energy performance from the databases in Table 2.2 (including split by ventilation type, where known)

2.5 HOW DO 'GREEN' OFFICE BUILDINGS PERFORM?

Figure 2.8 provides a summary of whole building annual energy consumption for a selection of 'green' buildings. These are buildings which have BREEAM ratings, have won sustainability awards or have been cited in books or journals as exemplar case studies. Appendix C provides an overview of each building's green credentials, the sources of data used and the assumptions made to convert the data to the $kgCO_2e$ per

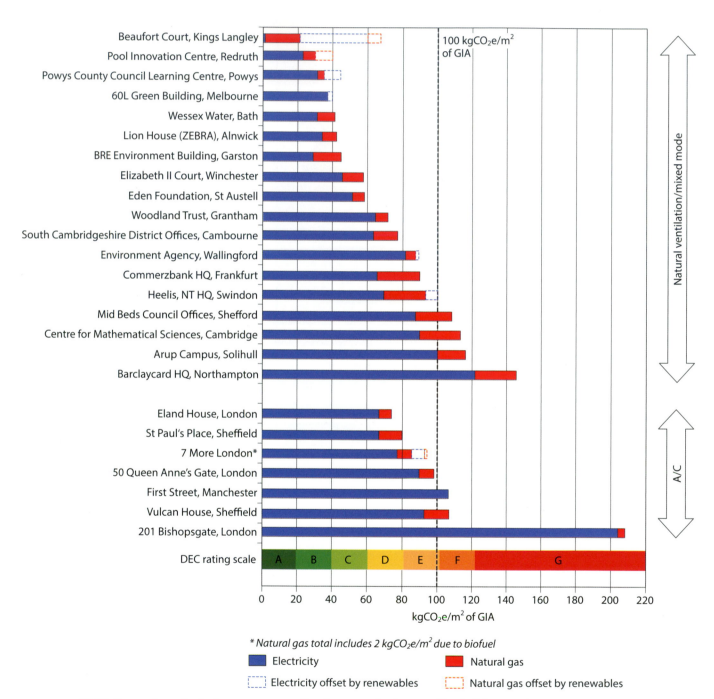

Fig 2.8 Comparison of actual energy consumption for a sample of green office buildings against the proposed 100 $kgCO_2e/m^2$ of GIA benchmark (refer to Appendix C for data sources and assumptions)

m^2 of GIA metric used throughout this book. The buildings are categorised as either 'air conditioned' (no openable windows) or 'mixed mode/naturally ventilated', and no attempt has been made to make adjustments for energy uses that might be excluded in formal energy ratings (e.g. regional data centres).

Reviewing the limited data in Figure 2.8 suggests that:

- a green design rating does not necessarily lead to a low-energy building
- air conditioned green offices tend to have higher energy consumption than those with an ability to naturally ventilate (consistent with the typical offices in Figure 2.7).

The majority of the best performing buildings in Figure 2.8 are between two and three storeys high and not located in busy city centres. Out-of-town offices tend to have the land area available to allow narrower floor plates (which enable effective daylighting and natural cross-ventilation) and fewer noise-related constraints on the use of openable windows. While out-of-town locations may lead to lower energy consumption, the issue of how people commute to these offices compared to city centre buildings, and the contribution this makes to the whole carbon footprint, is an issue that should not be ignored. This is discussed further in Chapters 4 and 5.

'People in glass ~~houses~~ offices shouldn't throw stones!'

Very few building owners publish the actual energy consumption of individual named buildings. The fact that the buildings in Figure 2.8 have publically released real performance data is to the great credit of their owners. It is also important to state here that the sole intention of showing the published data of the buildings is to put current energy benchmarks into perspective. It is not to criticise any of the buildings or to say that one is better than another, and this should not be inferred in any way from Figure 2.8. The data shown may not represent the current performance of these buildings and there is insufficient information available on hours of use, occupancy density, types of activity and climate during the year of the published energy data, to make detailed comparisons and to pass judgement. What should be evident, however, is that most of the green buildings in Figure 2.8 do perform better than the typical offices shown in Figure 2.7.

LEED BUILDINGS AND ENERGY CONSUMPTION

In 2008, a study of LEED rated buildings in the USA was undertaken.[18] Of the 552 buildings certified by 2006, 121 provided operating energy performance data, showing energy use that was 25–30% better than the national average (the Energy Star average in 2004 was 136 $kgCO_2e/m^2$). This suggests that LEED rated buildings would typically have an operating energy performance of around 100 $kgCO_2e/m^2$. The study also noted that a quarter of the LEED rated buildings performed more poorly than the average office building stock in the USA.

2.6 DESIGN ENERGY RATINGS VERSUS REALITY

Design energy modelling in the UK is usually limited to demonstrating compliance with Part L of the Building Regulations and calculating the Energy Performance Certificate (EPC) rating. This modelling provides a measure of energy efficiency of the building fabric and some, but not all, of the building services compared to a compliant base case building. It indicates the potential for the building to be low carbon, but has little or no correlation with actual performance.

Figure 2.9 summarises some office case study data from the CarbonBuzz website[19] which shows that metered energy consumption in a building can be over five times greater than the regulated design energy estimate. Figure 2.10 summarises a

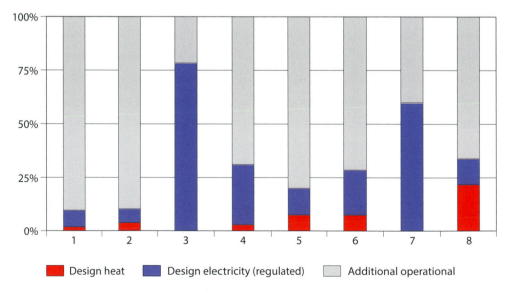

Fig 2.9 The proportion of design (EPC) estimates compared to actual energy consumption in eight UK office buildings (source: adapted from data on www.carbonbuzz.com)

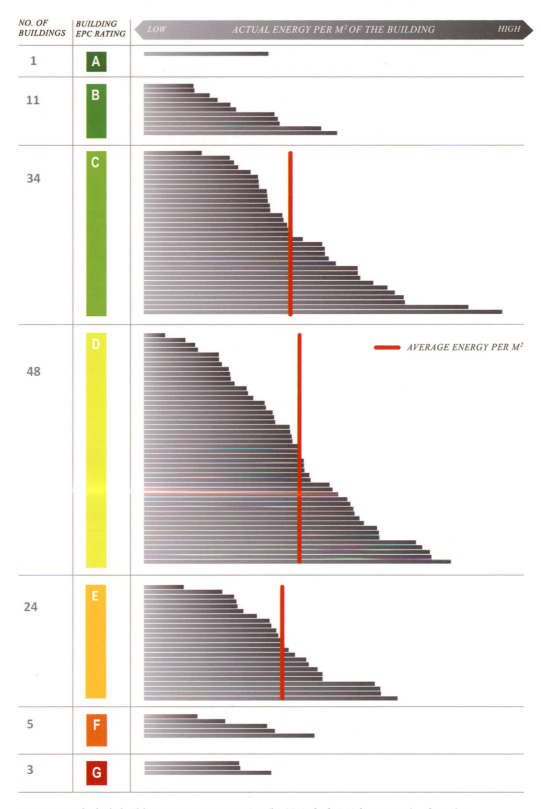

NO. OF BUILDINGS	BUILDING EPC RATING	LOW ──── ACTUAL ENERGY PER M² OF THE BUILDING ──── HIGH
1	A	
11	B	
34	C	
48	D	
24	E	
5	F	
3	G	

— AVERAGE ENERGY PER M²

Fig 2.10 Actual whole building energy consumption (kgCO$_2$/m² of NLA) for a sample of London office buildings grouped by EPC rating (source: Jones Lang LaSalle / Better Building Partnership, 2012)

CAREFUL DRIVING (OF BUILDINGS) SAVES ENERGY

Rating tools themselves do not save energy. Their purpose is to make energy visible and easy to understand in order to motivate occupants and building managers to act. Most of us understand that a car with a fuel consumption of 80 mpg (3.5 l/100 km) is economical and one with fuel consumption of 20 mpg (14 l/100 km) is not. We also know that how often we fill up the car depends on a number of factors, not just engine size. Table 2.3 shows a crude comparison of the factors affecting fuel economy in a car and the corresponding factors in a building.

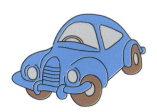
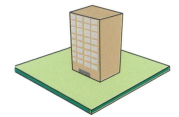

Engine size	Class of office
Number of seats	Floor area
Number of passengers carried	Occupant density
Luggage in boot or on roof	Servers and other special loads
Distance driven	Hours of occupancy
Careful and smooth driving	Energy management
Tyres and maintenance	Maintenance
Engine tuning	Recommissioning systems
Fuel gauge visible	Energy meters hidden in a cupboard

Table 2.3 Comparison of fuel economy factors in a car and a building

study by the Better Buildings Partnership (BBP) of 126 London office buildings in 2011, which found little or no correlation between the EPC rating and actual energy performance.[20] This shows almost no difference in median performance between C, D and E rated buildings, and some of the F and G rated buildings had lower energy consumption than the B rated buildings.

Part L energy modelling is used in BREEAM ratings and, from 2018, landlords in the UK will not be able to lease properties with an F or G rated EPC.[21] However, Part L and EPCs do not, and were never intended to, predict energy consumption in buildings. Unfortunately this is not widely appreciated and the $kgCO_2/m^2$ value from the computer output is often quoted as the predicted energy consumption of the building. Many building owners then get a surprise when the energy bills are much higher and the Display Energy Certificate (DEC) rating, based on actual performance, comes out as a 'G'. This is one reason why DECs are so rarely undertaken in the private sector. The performance gap between EPC and reality is discussed further in Chapter 6.

While EPCs undoubtedly have a role to play in improving the fabric of buildings and the energy efficiency of services, their limitations need to be understood if they are to usefully inform design decisions in new and refurbished buildings. They are not, however, the key tool to benchmark and drive actual reductions in the energy consumption and CO_2e emissions of real buildings.

2.7 THE NEED FOR SIMPLE, ROBUST ENERGY BENCHMARKS

If the commercial property sector is to make a meaningful contribution to reducing CO_2e emissions, a certified energy rating scheme that benchmarks real (not design) energy consumption consistently and fairly, and recognises incremental improvement in existing building stock, is a fundamental requirement. This should also reflect who controls the energy – landlord or tenants – and assess them individually as well as collectively.

Such a rating system can then be used to drive improvements through:

- providing transparent, robust benchmarks to compare performance with peers
- marketing of a building's performance to potential tenants
- inclusion of performance requirements in green leases or other contractual arrangements between landlord and tenants
- inclusion in new building or refurbishment contracts of a requirement for designers and contractors to deliver measured energy performance
- potentially linking energy ratings to taxation incentives.[22]

Appendix D proposes a modified rating methodology for UK office buildings, based on the existing Display Energy Certificate (DEC), with the following key attributes:

- a benchmark of 100 $kgCO_2e/m^2$ of GIA[23]
- adjustments for hours of use, occupancy density and unoccupied floors
- a rating scale to better reflect the diversity of energy performance across the commercial office sector and to encourage incremental improvement in existing building stock (see Figure 2.11)

- separate landlord and tenant benchmarks,[24] adjusted to suit the building services connected to the landlord and tenant meters:
  - landlord: 50 kgCO$_2$e/m^2
  - tenant: 750 kgCO$_2$e/person

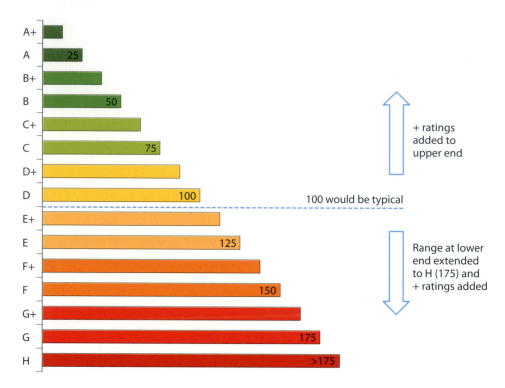

Fig 2.11 Potential energy rating scale for UK commercial office buildings?

2.8 SUMMARY

The primary purpose of an energy benchmark or rating is to make energy visible and to draw a line in the sand so that building owners, facility managers and occupants can put the energy consumption of their building into perspective – and then be motivated to take steps to reduce it. While this may sound simple, it is also apparent that without legislation there is currently little incentive for landlords and occupants to voluntarily report and display the annual energy performance of commercial buildings. To trot out the old cliché: if you don't measure it, you can't manage it.

In this chapter an **operating carbon benchmark for UK office buildings of 100 kgCO$_2$/m^2 of GIA** is proposed based on the emission factors used in Chapter 1. In addition to setting an appropriate benchmark, energy rating tools for operational buildings need to:

- be based on metered energy consumption because most design ratings have little correlation with actual performance
- make adjustments based on the intensity of use (occupancy density, hours of use and empty floors)
- use a rating scale which reflects the diversity of energy use in commercial buildings
- include separate benchmarks for landlords and tenants based on the energy they control and the building services they provide.

The very best performing green offices have an energy performance of between 30 and 40 $kgCO_2e/m^2$. They are typically owner occupied, two to four storeys tall, have openable windows and are located away from city centres. The majority of air conditioned commercial offices in the UK, which are possibly also more intensively occupied than the exemplar green buildings, rarely have an energy performance less than 100 $kgCO_2e/m^2$ of GIA and some exceed 200 $kgCO_2e/m^2$.

To get anywhere near zero carbon buildings in the future will require new technologies, lower carbon energy sources and, possibly the hardest nut to crack, changing the expectations and behaviour of the people designing, constructing, selling, managing and occupying buildings. While a step change in performance may be a while in coming, there are lots of opportunities to make significant reductions in energy use in most new and existing buildings today without too much difficulty. The starting point is to have a clear understanding of the actual performance, and how and where the energy is being used. Chapter 6 outlines ten steps to reducing energy consumption.

TO A/C OR NOT TO A/C? THAT IS A QUESTION

Air conditioning is associated with quality and comfort in commercial buildings, and therefore with higher rents and building value. It can also use a lot of energy. While not every building can be naturally ventilated, if offices in the future are to become 'nearly zero energy' then reducing reliance on mechanical systems to provide year-round comfort is an issue that needs to be addressed. At the very least, legislation could make it difficult to construct new buildings without openable windows, so that people can have the choice to switch off the air conditioning and open the windows (either now or in the future). Cars have heating, cooling and fresh air supply systems – but would you buy a car which didn't let you wind the windows down?

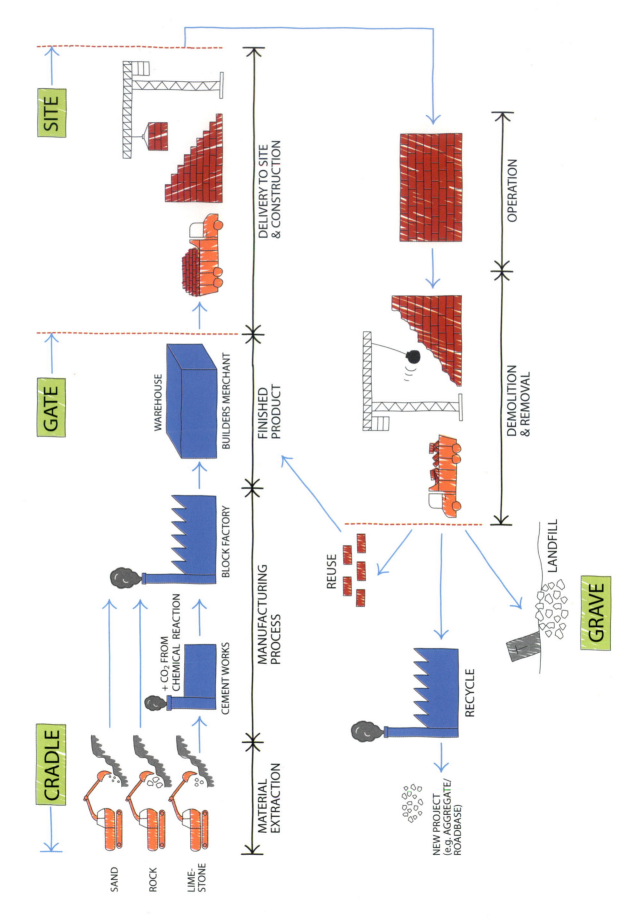

Fig 3.1 The embodied carbon stages in the life of a concrete block

materials. One of the most widely referenced sources of data in the UK, which is also freely available, is the *Inventory of Carbon and Energy* (ICE) developed by the University of Bath.[1]

Figure 3.1 shows the typical boundaries used in embodied carbon calculations. Different boundaries give different answers, so it is important to understand which one is being used:

- **Cradle**: this is the earth, or more specifically, the material deposits within or on the ground.
- **Cradle-to-gate**: the energy/carbon up to the factory gate of the final material/product.
- **Cradle-to-site**: cradle-to-gate plus delivery to the installation site (i.e. the building).
- **Cradle-to-grave**: the total processes from cradle to end of life.

Most embodied carbon factors for materials are published using cradle-to-gate boundaries.

3.2 CALCULATING THE EMBODIED CARBON OF INITIAL CONSTRUCTION

An embodied carbon assessment is basically a bill of quantities using carbon rates instead of cost rates. The first step is to calculate the total quantity of different materials and then multiply each by the relevant ECO_2 factor to obtain cradle-to-gate values. To estimate the cradle-to-site value, allowance must be made for site and fabrication wastage, transportation from the factory gate to the site and construction activities associated with installing the material or product. This can add between 5 to 20% to the total, the high variability due to the type of materials used, where they are sourced from and the level of site activity. All the values for each material or product are added together to give the total for the building. This process is summarised in Figure 3.3 (see page 51).

The ECO_2 factors adopted in the calculation have a very significant impact on the results. There is no industry standard approach and wide differences in values can be found.[2] Embodied carbon assessments should therefore really be expressed as a range to reflect uncertainties in data, rather than as an absolute value.

(FOOD) LABELLING OF BUILDING PRODUCTS

The majority of ECO$_2$ factors are based on generic or typical materials and products. To aid the selection of low-carbon products it would be useful if a similar approach to food labelling[3] (which has been mandatory and regulated for many years) was adopted.

If you want to select a low calorie (energy) material you could simply look at the label, which would also include other indicators such as embodied water, toxicity index, recycled content, recyclability and life expectancy. Labelling is critical to providing consumers with the information required to make an informed choice.

Some manufacturers do publish data on the environmental performance of their products but these are highly variable in scope and boundaries, making comparison between similar products difficult. New standards for the life cycle assessment and certification of products,[4] such as the EU's Environmental Product Declarations, should assist in delivering consistent, audited data in the future. However, these are currently voluntary and open to interpretation.

Servings per Package: 1	Average quantity	
Serving size: 170g	Per serving	Per 100g
Energy	410kJ	240kJ
Protein	5.2g	3.1g
Fat - total	4.8g	1.7g
- Saturated fat	0g	0g
Carbohydrate	11.5g	6.7g
- Sugars	3.5g	2.1g
Dietary fibre	2.2g	1.3g
Sodium	30mg	17mg
Potassium	335mg	210mg
Gluten	0mg	0mg
Iron	2.0mg	1.2mg

Typical food label

Standard:	EN _____	
Unit size:	___m² / m³ / kg	
Length of warranty:	___ years	
	Per kg	Per unit
Energy (MJ)		
Carbon (kgCO$_2$e)		
Water (litres)		
Recycled content (%)		
Recyclability (%)		
Non-renewable resources (%)		
VOC emissions		
Formaldehyde emissions		
Acidification potential		
Ozone depletion potential		
Global warming potential		
Toxicity rating		

Building product label?

Fig 3.2 A simple consumer label for building products?

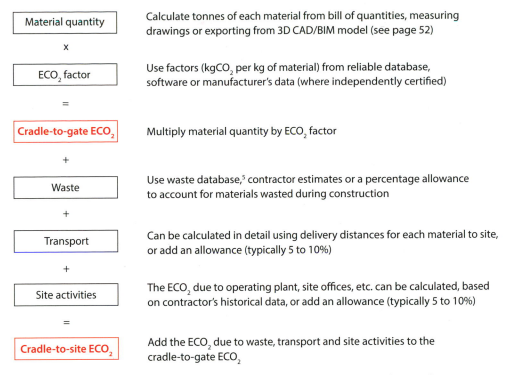

Material quantity	Calculate tonnes of each material from bill of quantities, measuring drawings or exporting from 3D CAD/BIM model (see page 52)
x	
ECO$_2$ factor	Use factors (kgCO$_2$ per kg of material) from reliable database, software or manufacturer's data (where independently certified)
=	
Cradle-to-gate ECO$_2$	Multiply material quantity by ECO$_2$ factor
+	
Waste	Use waste database,[5] contractor estimates or a percentage allowance to account for materials wasted during construction
+	
Transport	Can be calculated in detail using delivery distances for each material to site, or add an allowance (typically 5 to 10%)
+	
Site activities	The ECO$_2$ due to operating plant, site offices, etc. can be calculated, based on contractor's historical data, or add an allowance (typically 5 to 10%)
=	
Cradle-to-site ECO$_2$	Add the ECO$_2$ due to waste, transport and site activities to the cradle-to-gate ECO$_2$

Fig 3.3 **Typical process to calculate the embodied carbon of a building material or product**

3.3 SELECTING A LOW CARBON SOLUTION

The most important aspect of calculating the embodied carbon, irrespective of the methodology used, is to obtain the breakdown by materials or elements for a particular building. This can then be used to identify and target the biggest opportunities to reduce embodied carbon. The embodied carbon split for the construction of a new office building might look something like Figure 3.4. While the breakdown between different buildings is highly variable, the structure usually accounts for over half of the initial embodied carbon.

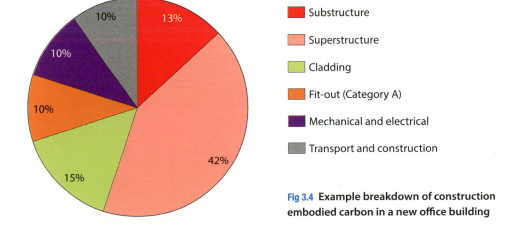

- Substructure
- Superstructure
- Cladding
- Fit-out (Category A)
- Mechanical and electrical
- Transport and construction

Fig 3.4 **Example breakdown of construction embodied carbon in a new office building**

BIM AND EMBODIED CARBON

The increasing use of 3D CAD and Building Information Modelling (BIM) from the schematic design stage of projects onwards will make it easier to determine the quantities of primary building materials, such as steel and concrete. By taking this information, and applying relevant ECO_2 factors, the embodied carbon of different design options and material specifications can be quickly compared.

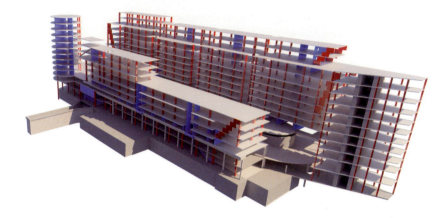

Fig 3.5 **Example 3D BIM structural schematic model**

For example, in the building model in Figure 3.5, the total volume of new reinforced concrete floor slab is 13,924 m³, with a total floor area of 56,613 m². To reduce the embodied carbon of concrete, the quantity of Portland cement needs to be reduced. Options include reducing the strength grade and increasing the quantity of cement replacements, such as ground granulated blast-furnace slag (GGBS) or pulverised fly ash (PFA). Table 3.1 illustrates the potential embodied carbon savings in the floor slabs due to a relatively minor change in the concrete mix specification compared to the base case. Further details on reducing the embodied carbon of concrete are provided in Chapter 8.

	Base	Option 1	Option 2	Option 3
Concrete grade	32/40	32/40	28/35	28/35
Cement replacement	15% PFA	25% GGBS	15% PFA	25% GGBS
$kgCO_2e$/tonne	152	133	138	119
$kgCO_2e$/m³	372	326	338	292
Total tCO_2e	**5,185**	**4,537**	**4,707**	**4,060**
$kgCO_2e$/m²	92	80	83	72
Saving tCO_2e	**–**	**648**	**478**	**1,126**
% saving	–	12%	9%	22%

Table 3.1 **Potential ECO_2 savings in concrete floor slab due to different concrete mixes**

It should be noted that the material or product with the lowest cradle-to-gate ECO_2 factor may not necessarily have the lowest carbon footprint over the life of the building. This is because materials and products have different properties (which affects the amount of material required to perform a function), durability (how often they need to be replaced over the design life of the building) and recyclability (what happens at the end of life).

There have been many studies undertaken to demonstrate the benefit of one material compared to another. The steel industry in the UK has been particularly active in advocating steel structures as being a lower embodied carbon solution in comparison to concrete and sometimes timber. This is discussed further in Chapter 8 and, without wishing to spoil the surprise, the author's conclusion is that there is very little difference between an efficiently designed steel structure and a concrete one.

3.4 EMBODIED CARBON OVER THE BUILDING LIFE

The typical design life of a new structure in the UK is assumed to be 60 years[6] although some stand for centuries and others are demolished after less than 20 years. While the structure may last 60 years, many components in a building, such as mechanical and electrical (M&E) plant, will be replaced or refurbished, often more than once, within this time frame. The most regularly replaced component is usually a tenant's fit-out – the majority of tenancy leases in the UK are less than 10 years, with almost half running for 5 years or less.[7] The process to calculate the embodied carbon for refurbishment and fit-out is the same as that described in Figure 3.3.

The whole life embodied carbon of a building is therefore a function of the initial embodied carbon, the life expectancy of the materials and equipment, the frequency of refurbishment and fit-out, how long the building lasts before it is pulled down and what happens to all the materials at the end of their life in the building. Various standards and methods have been, or are being, developed on carbon footprinting and embodied energy which aim to standardise the whole life calculation methodology.[8] Figure 3.6 (overleaf) shows the stages in the life of a typical building together with the corresponding life cycle modules A to C in European Standard EN 15978.[9]

The component of the whole life cycle that is probably most open to interpretation and uncertainty is the assumptions made regarding the disposal of a material at the end of its useful life in the building. Do you base the assumptions of what happens to the material on current typical practice (lots of demolition waste still goes to landfill), best practice (majority of materials recycled or reused) or some future, unknown technology/process (nothing goes to waste)? Module D of EN 15978 covers the reuse, recovery and/or recycling potential of materials separately as this is outside the building life cycle boundary.

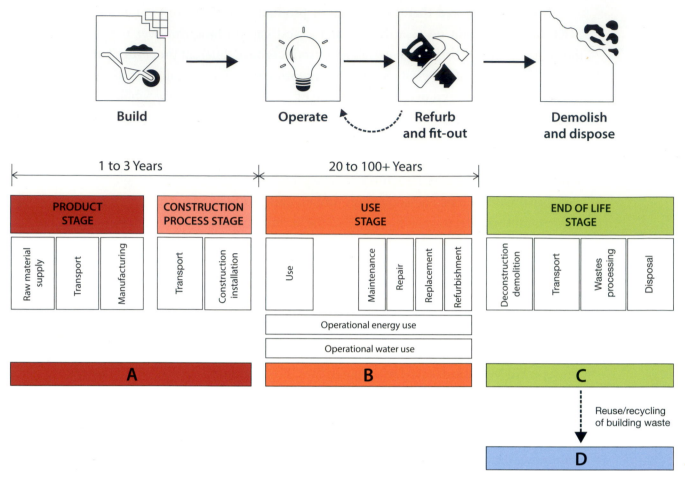

Fig 3.6 **The stages during the life of a typical building**
(and corresponding modules in EN 15978)

Different assumptions lead to significant differences in results. For example, does a steel structure have lower embodied carbon than a timber structure because the steel is recycled at the end of its life, while the timber may, or may not, end up as landfill and decompose releasing methane, which may, or may not, be captured for energy generation? Is a timber structure 'carbon negative' because the CO_2 absorbed by the trees is sequestered (stored) in the material? If the benefit of recycled steel is included in the initial construction ECO_2 factors, then should the benefit of recyclability at the end of life also be included, as this is counting the benefit twice?

The end-of-life assumptions can be highly contentious and must be clearly stated when calculating the whole life embodied carbon of a building.[10]

3.5 EMBODIED CARBON VALUES FROM CASE STUDIES

New construction

Figure 3.7 provides a summary of embodied carbon case studies for various office buildings.[11] The variation in values is due to the diversity of building stock assessed (height, materials, extent of basements, etc.), the extent of fit-out and finishes included in the

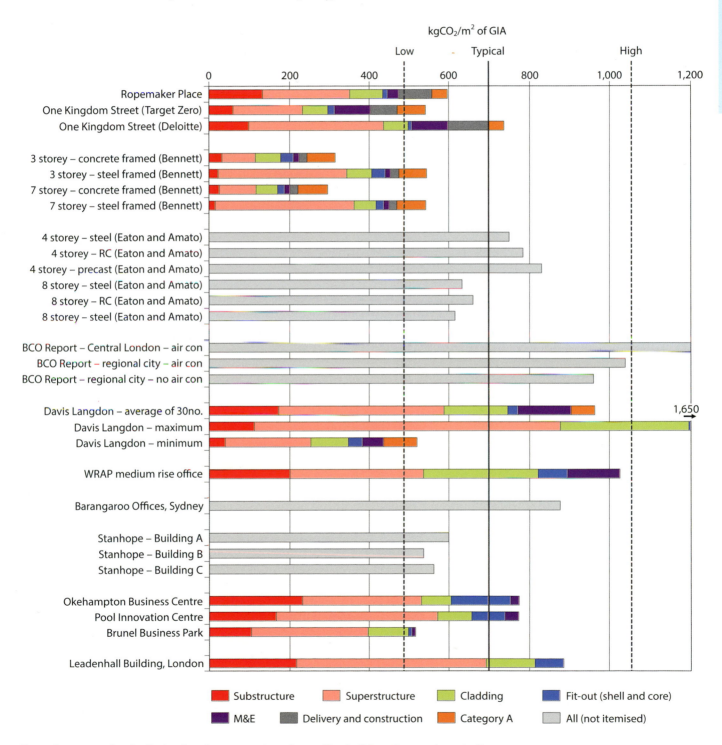

Fig 3.7 Summary of embodied carbon in construction of new office buildings from various studies

assessment, and the methodology used (system boundaries and ECO_2 factors adopted). While direct comparison between them is therefore not possible without detailed analysis of each assessment, what they do show is that the difference in values can be quite large, with extremes of 300 to 1,600 $kgCO_2/m^2$. The median of these various studies (counting the Davis Langdon average as a single study) is approximately 700 $kgCO_2/m^2$.

Office fit-out

In the UK, the British Council for Offices (BCO) *Guide to Specification*[12] separates the fit-out of office buildings into three categories: shell and core, Category A and Category B. The main components of an office fit-out are shown in Table 3.2. Some of these elements are undertaken by the landlord and some by the tenant.

Shell and core	Category A fit-out	Category B fit-out
Structure and façade	Raised floor	Partitions
Central plant and services	Ceiling	Joinery
Core finishes	Floor finishes	Furniture
(e.g. toilets, lift lobbies)	Tenant lighting	Supplementary tenant services
	HVAC (floor/ceiling)	(e.g. A/C to server room)

Table 3.2 **Typical components in fit-out of UK office buildings**

Most of the initial construction studies in Figure 3.7 did not separate shell and core and Category A fit-out elements and not all of the studies included carpets. Consideration of the data available, and adding in an allowance for carpets, suggests that a Category A fit-out might account for around **100 $kgCO_2/m^2$**.

There have been very few detailed studies undertaken to calculate the embodied carbon of a tenant (Category B) fit-out. Table 3.3 provides a summary of three sources of data, which suggests that a typical value for a Category B fit-out might be between **100 and 200 $kgCO_2e/m^2$**. If this occurs every 10 years then it could represent a significant proportion (up to 50%) of the whole life embodied carbon of a typical office building. Further research into the embodied carbon of fit-outs is clearly needed.

Source	ECO_2 values $(kgCO_2/m^2)$	Comments
Stanhope report[13]	98 to 212	Case studies of four Stanhope buildings in 2010. Scope of Category A and B fit-out not stated
WRAP case study[14]	190	A study by WRAP for a large office fit-out in an urban area
Appendix E	180 to 450	Estimated using input:output ECO_2 data $(kgCO_2/£)$ for fit-out costs between £500 and £1,250 per m^2

Table 3.3 **Embodied carbon values for tenant fit-out**

FIT-OUT VERSUS STRUCTURE

In the *Green Guide to Specification* (2002),[15] the Building Research Establishment (BRE) calculated the embodied environmental impacts for different building elements in a typical office building over a 60-year design life (including maintenance and replacement). The impacts, shown in Figure 3.8, were based on Ecopoints,[16] which combine 12 environmental issues into a single score. Climate change and fossil fuel depletion accounted for 50% of the relative weighting in an Ecopoint.

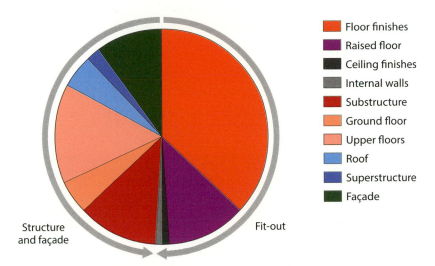

Floor finishes
Raised floor
Ceiling finishes
Internal walls
Substructure
Ground floor
Upper floors
Roof
Superstructure
Façade

Structure and façade

Fit-out

Fig 3.8 **Contribution of building elements to typical building impact** (adapted from BRE *Green Guide to Specification*, 2002)

The assessment assumed a wool/nylon carpet with foam underlay being replaced every 5 years and, based on this, carpet accounted for a staggering 40% of the total environmental impact over 60 years. Specifying lower impact, longer lasting carpets and not replacing them as regularly, saves carbon, waste, resource consumption and money. The second highest impact was the floor structure (15%) with raised access floors coming in a close third at 12%. So, according to this study, about half the environmental impact of the office building is associated with the flooring placed onto the floor slab. While the assumed frequency of carpet replacement might be excessive in many buildings, fit-out is clearly an important issue, but is not always included in embodied carbon assessments.

End of life

What happens to materials at the end of life is a complex issue. Various studies based on current demolition practices suggest that the site activities (energy consumption of plant and equipment) and waste transportation and disposal account for between 3 and 5% of the total embodied carbon (ignoring the benefits of recycling materials).[17]

3.6 TYPICAL EMBODIED CARBON VALUES FOR OFFICES

Table 3.4 shows indicative values assumed for the embodied carbon of a typical UK office building based on the studies shown in Figure 3.7. While every building is unique, the suggested values provide a simple rule of thumb for the purpose of putting the embodied and operating carbon contributions to the whole carbon footprint of an office building into perspective. The 'low carbon design' value represents a 33% reduction in the typical design, while the 'high carbon design' represents a 50% increase.

These values are *not* embodied carbon benchmarks as they are not drawn from a wide enough data set, have not been subjected to detailed scrutiny of boundary conditions, methodologies and ECO_2 factors used, and do not consider adjustments for basements, building heights and so on. Significant research is required to develop robust embodied carbon benchmarks for different building types.[18]

	Indicative embodied carbon values ($kgCO_2e/m^2$ of GIA)		
	Typical design	Low carbon design	High carbon design
New build (shell and core)	600	400	900
Fit-out (Category A)	100	70	150
New building total	**700**	**470**	**1,050**
Fit-out (Category B)*	200	100	300
Minor refurbishment (excluding fit-out)	25	15	40
Major refurbishment (excluding fit-out)	100	70	150
Reclad	100	70	150
Demolition and disposal	30	30	30

* The values for Category B fit-out have a high degree of uncertainty due to minimal data being available.

Table 3.4 **Indicative embodied carbon values for UK office buildings**

3.7 EMBODIED VERSUS OPERATING CARBON IN OFFICE BUILDINGS

The relative importance of embodied versus operating carbon over the life of a building can prompt a lot of debate. To allow transparent comparisons to be made for different scenarios, the assumptions shown in Table 3.5 are used to establish a base case building over 60 years. Category B fit-out is excluded due to the lack of reliable benchmarking data.

	$kgCO_2e/m^2$ of GIA	Frequency	Total $kgCO_2e/m^2$ over 60 years
New building (shell and core)	600	Year 1	600
Category A fit-out (four times)	100	Years 1, 15, 30 & 45	400
Minor refurbishment (twice)	25	Years 15 & 45	50
Major refurbishment	100	Year 30	100
Total embodied carbon			**1,150**
Operating energy for whole building[19]	100	Years 2 to 29	2,800
Operating energy after major refurbishment	70	Years 31 to 60	2,100
Total operating carbon			**4,900**

Table 3.5 Base case assumptions for embodied v operating carbon assessment

While the energy consumption and emissions will vary over time, for the base case, no changes in the values over the 60-year period are assumed, except after the major refurbishment in year 30, when the operating energy reduces by 30% due to replacement with more energy efficient plant. What happens to the building after 60 years is excluded from this comparison.

Figure 3.9 (overleaf) shows the emissions each year based on the base case assumptions. Figure 3.10 (overleaf) shows the cumulative carbon emissions, with the initial embodied carbon due to construction representing 12% of the total over a 60-year lifespan. This is equivalent to about 7 years of operating energy.

The base case ignored the Category B fit-out. If a value of 200 $kgCO_2e/m^2$ were assumed, and the Category B fit-out occurred every 10 years, then its carbon footprint would be approximately 20 $kgCO_2e/m^2$ per year. The embodied carbon due to the Category B fit-out could be as large as the initial construction, refurbishment and Category A fit-outs combined.

The base case assessment was based on the assumptions in Table 3.5. Figure 3.11 shows how the results vary based on the scenarios shown in Table 3.6 (page 61). The

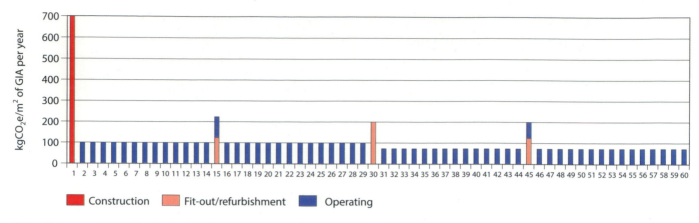

Fig 3.9 Base case – annual embodied and operating carbon (kgCO$_2$e/m^2)

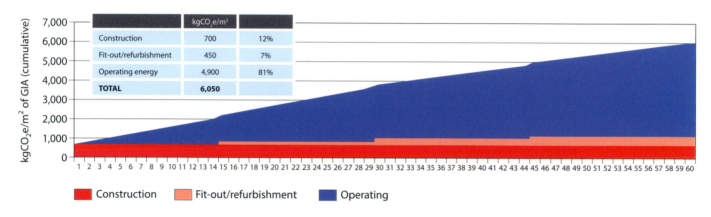

Fig 3.10 Base case – cumulative embodied v operating carbon (kgCO$_2$e/m^2 of GIA)

base case and scenarios 1 to 3 were all based on the current UK grid electricity emission factor. Scenario 4 considers the impact on the operating and embodied carbon due to grid electricity supplied from less carbon-intensive sources, such as renewables and nuclear. Further details, calculated values and individual graphs (similar to Figure 3.10) for each scenario are given in Appendix E.

This analysis shows that variations in operating energy have a much greater influence on the whole carbon footprint than variations in embodied carbon. Reducing the energy consumption of buildings is therefore still the highest priority, but the two are not mutually exclusive. Reducing the embodied carbon of the initial construction, fit-out and refurbishments will provide clear benefits, often at little or no capital cost.

A perhaps surprising result, based on the assumptions made, was that knocking the building down after 30 years and replacing it with a more energy efficient version, showed little difference (+/- 8%) compared to the base case of a building standing for 60 years. However, this does not take into consideration any of the other environmental impacts of such a strategy, including waste generation and depletion of natural resources – carbon is not the only factor to consider.

	Variable	Assumption
1	**Embodied carbon**	
	(a) Low ECO$_2$	33% reduction compared to base case (refer Table 3.4)
	(b) High ECO$_2$	50% increase compared to base case (refer Table 3.4)
2	**Operating energy**	
	(a) Low energy	33% reduction compared to base case
	(b) High energy	50% increase compared to base case
3	**Rebuild after 30 years**	New building in Year 1, knock down and rebuild in Year 30
	(a) Base case	Replacement has same efficiency as base case refurbished building
	(b) Low energy	Replacement is 60% more efficient (40 kgCO$_2$e/m^2)
4	**Grid decarbonisation**	Reduction in kgCO$_2$e/kWh emissions factor for grid electricity
	(a) Best case	80% by 2050 and 90% by 2070
	(b) Political reality?	45% by 2050 and 75% by 2070

Table 3.6 Different scenarios for embodied v operating carbon comparison

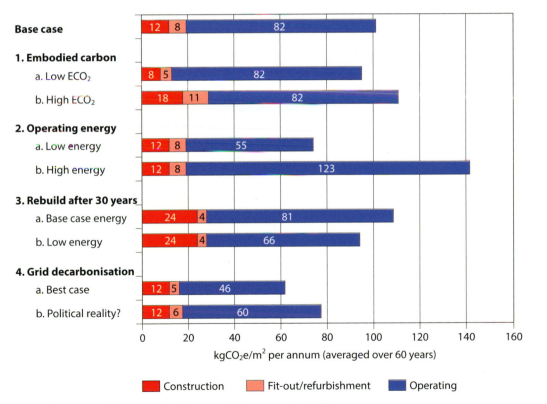

Fig 3.11 Summary of four scenarios for embodied v operating carbon

Figure 3.11 shows that the biggest influence over 60 years is the proposed decarbonisation of the electricity grid, which is outside the control of the builder, the building owner and the occupants. In the best case decarbonisation scenario, the embodied carbon of the initial construction would account for 26% of the whole carbon footprint (compared to 12% in the base case). Under this scenario, and with the structure accounting for around half of this, structural engineers are in a position to influence the components contributing to around 10% of the carbon footprint.

To conclude the assessment, a combination of the scenarios to obtain realistic upper and lower values for the operating and embodied carbon footprint of a typical office building over 60 years were considered:

- lower bound scenario = 1a + 2a + 4a
- upper bound scenario = 1b + 2b + 4b.

The results in Figure 3.12 show that the difference between the two scenarios is almost a factor of 3, with the upper limit not much more than the base case when some grid decarbonisation over the next 60 years is included. The embodied carbon in the initial construction represents 19% of the lower total and 15% of the upper total.

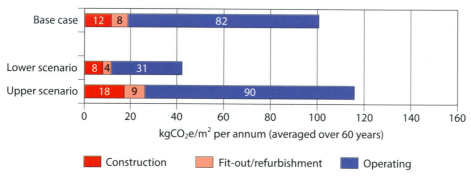

Fig 3.12 **Summary of upper and lower bound decarbonisation scenarios for embodied v operating carbon**

3.8 SUMMARY

Embodied carbon is the CO_2e emissions due to the construction, refurbishment and demolition of buildings. The embodied carbon for new construction of office buildings is typically between 500 and 900 $kgCO_2e/m^2$ of GIA. This is equivalent to 5 to 10 years of the CO_2e emissions due to the energy consumption of typical UK office buildings.

Sometimes embodied carbon is compared to regulated design energy, which would suggest that it is equivalent to 28 years of operating carbon.[20] This is because, as shown in Chapter 2, design energy can be up to 5 times less than actual energy consumption. If embodied carbon assessments are intended to estimate the actual CO_2e emissions due to construction, then they should really be compared with the CO_2e emissions due to actual operation.

Embodied carbon is clearly important, but it is not as significant as energy consumption. It does, however, represent the first CO_2 emissions associated with a building and, once released, cannot be taken back (with operating carbon there is always the opportunity to make reductions at any time over the life of the building).

Agreeing how to measure whole life embodied carbon is still problematic, but reducing it through resource efficiency (good design and material specification) is relatively straightforward. The embodied carbon due to fit-out is not well understood, but could account for up to half of the whole life embodied carbon and this warrants further research.

Undertaking a detailed assessment of embodied carbon is often expensive, but rules of thumb are just as useful in the early stages of design when key decisions are being made. The structure typically represents around half the initial construction carbon, but due to the wide range of data and assumptions for different structural materials, embodied carbon assessment is not a reliable tool for deciding the structural form. This is discussed further in Chapter 8.

Once a structural form or material is chosen, the next step is to choose or specify a low-carbon version. The increasing use of 3D CAD and BIM should make estimating the embodied carbon of the structural and façade elements relatively straightforward during design development, enabling reductions due to different material and specification options to be quickly tested.

One of the best ways in which designers and contractors can reduce embodied carbon is to challenge the supply chain to deliver lower carbon products. While the building industry can be notoriously conservative and slow to innovate, the power of purchasers to influence a market should not be underestimated. Reliable and transparent product labelling will be essential to facilitate this.

Voluntary action alone is unlikely to be sufficient to propel the property industry along a low embodied carbon path and some form of embodied carbon legislation may be introduced in the future.[21] In the meantime, rating tools may encourage some developers and contractors to measure embodied carbon. For example, Germany's DGNB rating tool uses life cycle assessment of operating and embodied energy and awards points based on primary energy demand and CO_2 emissions. In BREEAM and LEED, operating and embodied energy are assessed separately under energy and materials categories.[22] Surprisingly, unlike BREEAM and LEED, the location of the building, and how people travel to it, isn't included in the final DGNB rating score. How important is location? The contribution of transport emissions to the whole carbon footprint is covered in the next chapter.

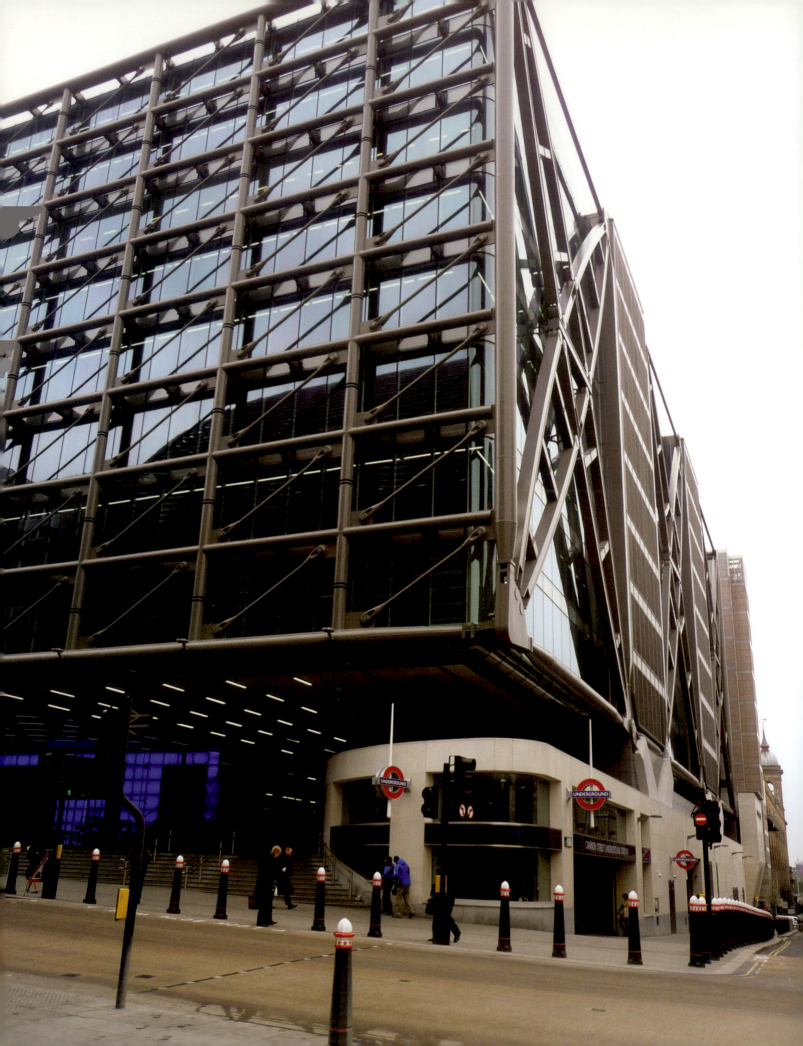

Chapter 4

Transport carbon

I got rid of the Ferrari: it was bad for my hamstrings.
Ryan Giggs, Manchester United FC

The operating and embodied carbon due to the design, construction and operation of office buildings was discussed in Chapters 2 and 3. However, transport is rarely given much emphasis when considering the whole energy and carbon footprint of buildings. This chapter looks at how people commute to and from UK offices, the CO_2e emissions associated with commuting and the influence that location has on a building's carbon footprint. Business travel[1] is excluded as this will vary significantly with the nature of the businesses in the building.

4.1 UK TRANSPORT EMISSIONS IN CONTEXT

In 2011, emissions due to transport amounted to 119 million tCO_2e, between 20 to 25% of the UK's total CO_2e emissions.[2] Transport emissions have now returned to around 1990 levels after peaking in 2007, although the reduction since then may have been influenced in part by the global economic downturn that started in 2008. Figure 4.1 (overleaf) shows the breakdown of CO_2e emissions by transport type in 2011.

Figure 4.2 (overleaf) shows the breakdown of distance travelled for commuting and business purposes in 2010.[3] Cars and motorcycles account for three-quarters of the distance travelled for commuting and business purposes. Since 1990, the annual distance travelled by car in the UK (for business and personal use) has remained relatively consistent at around 11,000 km per person.[4]

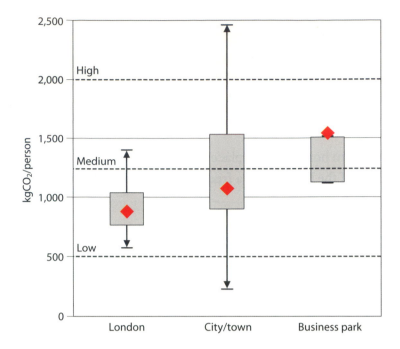

The grey blocks show the survey results falling within the upper and lower quartiles.
The vertical lines show the full range of results.
The diamonds show the results of the 2002 census data analysis. (Source: Wyatt, P.)

Fig 4.3 **Summary of commuting survey results and 2002 census analysis by location type**

Cundall's Birmingham office (2,358 $kgCO_2$/person) was the highest, despite being reasonably close to the city centre. The respondents to the survey in this office showed that cars accounted for 77% of the distance travelled (representing over 90% of the CO_2 emissions from travel) because a number of staff live outside Birmingham and the local rail-based public transport system is not as extensive as in other cities.

This highlights one of the major difficulties with predicting transport emissions – the distance and mode of travel is a major variable. It depends on where people live and cannot be reliably estimated by only considering a building's proximity to public transport, car parking provision and the number of bike racks provided. These are the criteria used by most rating tools to score transport points.

4.4 TRANSPORT ASSESSMENTS

To determine travel CO_2e emissions in occupied buildings, travel surveys can be undertaken. To estimate the emissions in new or unoccupied buildings is not so simple. One method could be to use Transport Assessments. These are usually a requirement for planning applications for new office buildings in the UK. While their purpose is primarily to identify issues with traffic congestion and parking, the data can be used to make crude estimates of annual travel distances and transport modes and, consequently, CO_2e emissions. This is useful for speculative new offices, where the occupants' travel modes and distances are not known.

Appendix F outlines how statistical census data on travel to work distances and modes of transport was converted into $kgCO_2e$/person per annum estimates for four Cundall offices. The results, compared to the Cundall Travel Survey and indicative BREEAM 2011 transport scores, are summarised in Figure 4.4.

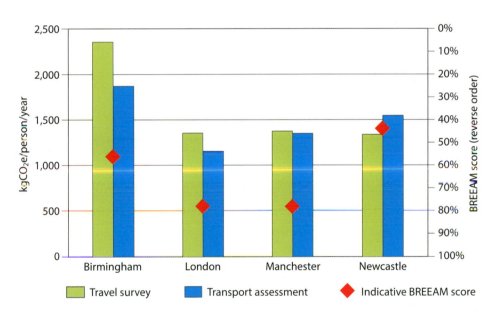

Fig 4.4 Comparison of survey results with Transport Assessments for Cundall UK offices

Statistical travel data could potentially be used to provide a simple method of estimating transport carbon during the planning and design stages of projects. There may also be some potential to incorporate this approach into rating tool assessments. Further research into how an office's geographic location, proximity to public transport and car parking, and provision of cycling facilities influence transport emissions is necessary to more accurately predict transport emissions prior to occupation.

4.5 TRANSPORT CARBON VERSUS OPERATING CARBON

To compare the transport emissions with operating and embodied carbon requires converting $kgCO_2e$/person into $kgCO_2e/m^2$ of GIA. This now introduces another variable that can distort the comparison between buildings – a near-empty building will have a much lower $kgCO_2e/m^2$ than a densely occupied one. Since we are only concerned with putting emissions into perspective at this stage, an average occupancy of one person per 15 m^2 of GIA will be adopted, which is consistent with the average occupancy density used in Chapter 2.

In this book, three categories for transport carbon are adopted, as shown in Table 4.1, to include in the review of the whole carbon footprint in the next chapter.

	$kgCO_2e$/person	$kgCO_2e/m^2$ of GIA
Low	500	33
Medium	1,250	83
High	2,000	133

Table 4.1 Comparative transport carbon values for UK office buildings

In Chapter 2, the typical operating carbon benchmark was proposed as 100 $kgCO_2e/m^2$ of GIA. The energy resource consumption and CO_2e emissions due to transport could therefore be higher than those due to operating energy in some office buildings. This might apply to many of the green offices in out-of-town locations in Figure 2.8 in Chapter 2. Various scenarios of operating versus embodied versus transport carbon are considered in Chapter 5.

4.6 SUMMARY

A review of the limited data available for travel associated with office buildings in the UK suggests that annual transport CO_2e emissions for commuting typically fall within a range between 750 and 1,500 $kgCO_2e$/person. Transport carbon can consequently be higher than operating carbon in some office buildings. The distance that people travel to work (and their mode of transport) is a major variable and difficult to predict at the planning and design stages. Transport Assessment data could potentially be used when actual occupant survey data is not available.

While transport carbon can be difficult to predict or quantify, particularly when planning new buildings, one thing is clear, the importance of a building's location should not be understated or ignored when considering its carbon footprint and credentials – but it usually is.

Chapter 9 provides guidance on how landlords and tenants can reduce CO_2e emissions due to commuting to and from office buildings.

THE FUTURE DECARBONISATION OF TRANSPORT?

In Chapter 3, the effect of grid decarbonisation on operating carbon over the next 60 years was considered. Under the UK Committee on Climate Change's medium abatement scenario it is estimated that it will be possible to reduce surface transport CO_2e emissions in 2030 by 44% relative to 2008 levels.[7] In comparison, over the same period the Committee estimates that building heating emissions can be reduced by 74% while the carbon intensity of grid electricity supplied to buildings needs to be reduced by 90%. This suggests that carbon reduction will be easier to achieve in building operation than in transport, and the proportion of transport emissions in a building's overall carbon footprint will therefore increase over time.

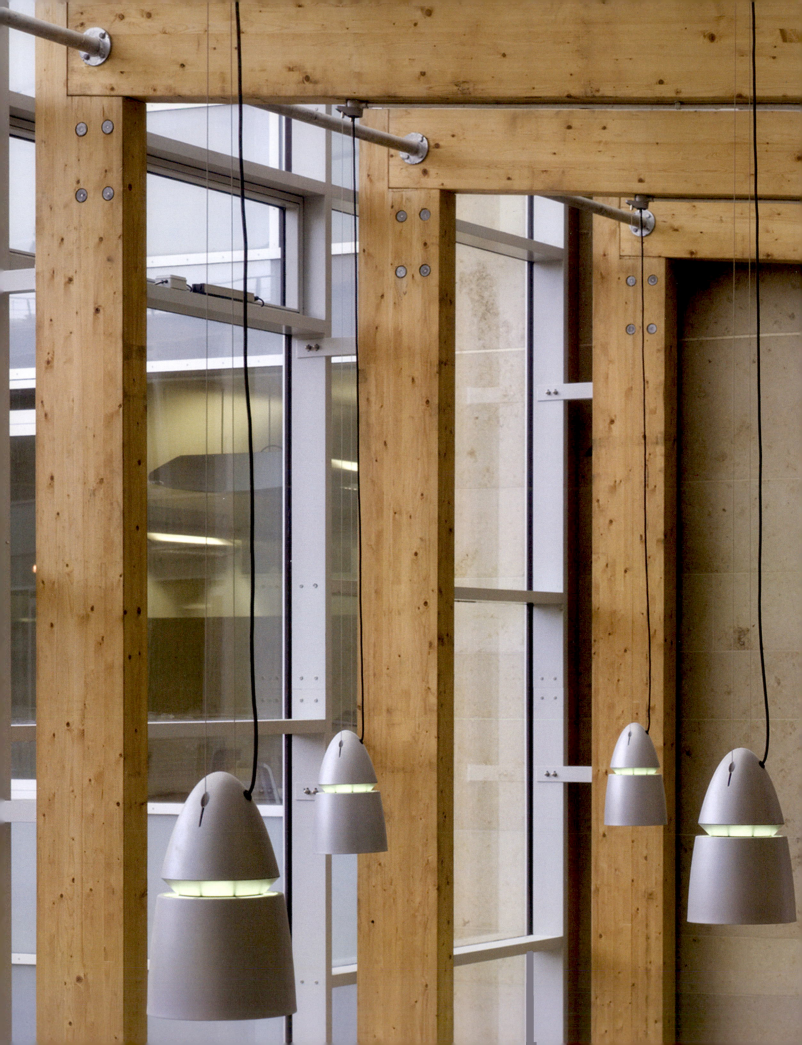

Chapter 5

Whole carbon footprint

Statistics are like a bikini. What they reveal is suggestive, but what they conceal is vital.

Aaron Levenstein, American economist

In the introduction to this book the whole carbon footprint (which is also a proxy for energy resource consumption) was defined as the greenhouse gas emissions associated with:

- **Operating energy** – the electricity, gas and other fuels used in a building for heating, cooling, ventilation, lighting, hot water, computers, servers and other equipment.
- **Embodied energy** – the energy consumed in manufacturing, delivering and installing the materials used to build, fit-out and refurbish a building.
- **Transport energy** – the energy used to get people to and from a building.

In Chapters 2, 3 and 4, the typical CO_2e emissions for each of these in office buildings was discussed. The final step is to combine them into a simple single metric that can be used to consider the whole energy and carbon footprint during the planning and design stages of projects and the operation of existing buildings.

5.1 DEVELOPING A SINGLE METRIC

The CO_2e emissions for operating, embodied and transport are in different formats (refer to Table 5.1 overleaf) and some assumptions need to be made to combine them into a single, comparable metric. Should the metric be based on floor area (m²) or occupancy (number of people)? What is the time period for evaluation of embodied

	Operating	Embodied	Transport
Measurement	$kgCO_2e/m^2/year$	$kgCO_2e/m^2$	$kgCO_2e/person/year$
Time period	1 year	60 years	1 year
Impact of future decarbonisation	Reduces carbon each year	No impact on initial construction. Some impact on fit-out/refurbishment	Reduces carbon each year

Table 5.1 Key differences between operating, embodied and transport carbon metrics

carbon? Should the predicted national decarbonisation of energy supply, manufacturing and transportation sectors over time be included?

The following assumptions will be adopted for the whole carbon footprint metric proposed in this book:

- The footprint will be based on 1 year of carbon emissions (with 2,600 typical hours of use).
- The unit will be $kgCO_2e/m^2$ of GIA with an assumed base occupancy of one person per 15 m^2.
- The annualised embodied carbon will be equal to the total calculated CO_2e emissions over 60 years divided by 60.
- The effect of decarbonisation will be excluded as it is difficult to predict this with any degree of certainty (and it will affect all three components to some degree anyway).

For each carbon component, three benchmark scenarios are considered: high, typical and low. The values are taken from the previous chapters and summarised in Table 5.2.

Figure 5.1 shows the breakdown of carbon in an office building with the typical operating, embodied and transport benchmarks. While every building will have its own unique footprint and breakdown, this diagram is useful in indicating the importance of the building location and commuting habits of the occupants on the overall carbon footprint.

	$kgCO_2e/m^2$ of GIA/year				
	Operating	Embodied (initial)	Embodied (refurbishment/ fit-out)	Transport	**Total**
Low	50	8	5	33	**96**
Typical	100	12	8	83	**203**
High	150	18	11	133	**312**

Table 5.2 Whole carbon footprint benchmarks for UK offices (excluding Category B fit-out)

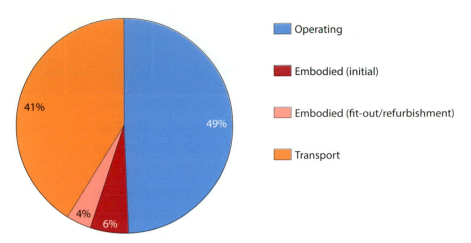

Fig 5.1 Carbon footprint breakdown of an office building in the UK using typical benchmarks for each category (excluding Category B fit-out)

In Chapter 3, the embodied carbon of a Category B fit-out was estimated to be between 100 and 200 $kgCO_2e/m^2$. A 200 $kgCO_2e/m^2$ fit-out every 10 years over a 60-year period is equivalent to 20 $kgCO_2e/m^2$ per annum, which represents an additional 10% on the typical whole carbon footprint. This is a subject where further research is required, but due to the uncertainty in current data it has been excluded from the whole carbon footprint calculations.

5.2 COMPARING PERFORMANCE AGAINST THE BENCHMARKS

Table 5.3 (overleaf) shows some hypothetical data for a range of office types and locations to illustrate the principle of the whole carbon footprint. The data for Cundall's existing UK offices is also shown with assumed embodied carbon data for future refurbishment and fit-out (as per Table 3.5 in Chapter 3).[1] Figure 5.2 shows the same buildings after converting the values into annual $kgCO_2e/m^2$ of GIA, but without any adjustment for occupancy density or hours of use.

This assessment illustrates that it is difficult to achieve a building that has low carbon emissions for all three categories: operating, embodied and transport. The majority of low energy green buildings in Figure 2.8 in Chapter 2 tend to be under four storeys with layouts that enable natural ventilation, daylight and on-site renewables to be utilised effectively. However, many of these are located in rural or edge-of-town locations and are therefore likely to have high transport emissions. The low operating carbon emissions of these buildings are rightly celebrated as exemplar,

PLANNING FOR LOW CARBON BUILDINGS

To obtain planning permission for a new building usually requires:

- a sustainability box to be ticked somewhere in the application (often by issuing a sustainability statement and installing 10% renewables)
- sufficient car parking spaces to be provided.

If we consider the 'hypothetical new air conditioned office in a business park' in Table 5.3 then, assuming it is built to 2010 UK Building Regulations, a 10% renewables target[3] for planning approval might require the installation of systems to reduce CO_2e emissions by 3 $kgCO_2e/m^2$. This represents less than 2% of the whole carbon footprint. To put this into context, the transport emissions in a business park are typically at least 20 $kgCO_2e/m^2$ higher than those in a city centre or town. The extra space available to install renewables on low-rise out-of-town buildings does not outweigh the increased transport emissions.

It could therefore be argued that buildings located away from public transport should have more stringent operating carbon standards imposed upon them than inner city buildings. While this sounds reasonable in principle, it raises a number of tricky questions. Where do you draw the boundary? Is it equitable, because although land is cheaper, rents outside city centres are also lower, which means there is less capital to spend on energy efficiency and renewables. And how can targets be established anyway when, as this book has already shown, there is such limited benchmarking data available?

Considering the whole carbon footprint, rather than just selected parts of it, will become increasingly important when making strategic decisions about the future built environment. A simple whole carbon footprint methodology (or rating tool) could be useful to inform decision making for both new and existing buildings.

Rating scales using letters (A to G), scores out of 100, descriptions (good to excellent), precious metals (bronze to platinum) and number of stars (or other objects) have all been used to create a simple indicator of performance. As long as the scale is clearly defined then the building's performance relative to the benchmark – good, average or poor – can be seen at a glance, without having to delve into the detail behind the calculations.

Appendix G describes a potential methodology for a simple whole carbon rating using the data and principles set out in this book. A basic tool using the methodology can be downloaded from **www.wholecarbonfootprint.com**. The rating score calculation is:

$$\text{Score} = \frac{\text{total footprint (kgCO}_2\text{e/m}^2) \times 100}{\text{adjusted benchmark (kgCO}_2\text{e/m}^2)}$$

The primary inputs required to benchmark a building are:

- floor area
- annual energy consumption
- embodied carbon over a 60-year period
- travel emissions per person per year
- occupancy density*
- hours of use*
- CO_2e emission factors for electricity and heating source*
- frequency of fit-out and refurbishment.

The benchmark is adjusted to suit variables marked with an asterisk (*) and default values for low, typical and high embodied and transport emissions can be used if actual values for a building are not known.

The rating is expressed as a score (where 0 is zero carbon and 100 is typical). This score is also converted to a letter and a number of stars to illustrate how the rating can be represented using different scales. Graphs showing the breakdown of the footprint are also provided. The methodology can be used for planning stage assessments, using typical values, or to benchmark actual buildings based on measured energy and CO_2e emissions.

Table 5.4 (overleaf) shows the ratings of five of Cundall's UK offices using the tool. The rating scores give different results to that which might be assumed if the operating carbon alone was used, or the benchmarks were not adjusted to reflect occupancy density. Figure 5.3 shows the rating score for each office compared to the score if it were calculated using benchmarks based only on area (kgCO$_2$e/m^2) or only on occupancy density (kgCO$_2$e/person).[4]

The rating score for each falls roughly midway between the unadjusted scores by area and by person. Taking occupancy density into account is clearly important for whole carbon footprint ratings otherwise the rating would penalise more densely occupied buildings. This also shows that, by using the same data, one building can be shown to be better or worse than another, depending on which approach is adopted. For example, the Edinburgh office was the lowest by floor area but not by person. Benchmarking energy and carbon performance in office buildings needs to take a balanced approach to avoid these discrepancies.

The methodology described in this chapter is not meant to be an official rating, but instead illustrates a simple method of comparing the whole carbon footprint of buildings to promote debate in the industry about how this should be considered in the planning, design and operation of buildings.

Cundall office	Carbon footprint (kgCO$_2$e/m²)	Adjusted benchmark (kgCO$_2$e/m²)	Score	Rating	Alternative star rating	tCO$_2$e/person
Birmingham	153	144	106	E+	2.5	3.8
Edinburgh	127	144	88	D	3	3.2
London	232	203	114	E	2	3.2
Manchester	139	147	94	D	3	3.3
Newcastle	194	209	93	D	3	2.6

Table 5.4 Cundall UK offices – whole carbon footprint ratings

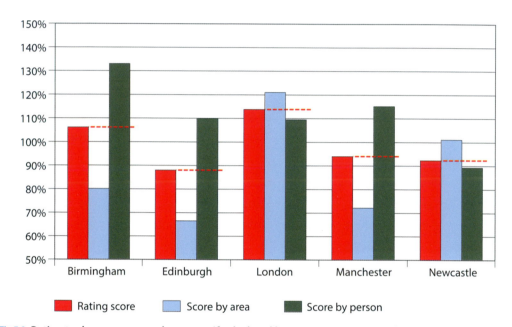

Fig 5.3 Rating tool score compared to scores if calculated by area or occupancy only

The methodology can be adapted for other building types and buildings outside the UK by:

- using different CO$_2$e emission factors (or converting to primary energy factors)
- setting appropriate benchmarks for operating, embodied and transport to suit the location and climate.

5.4 SUMMARY

The whole carbon footprint challenge for buildings is illustrated in Figure 5.4. We don't need low operating carbon or low transport carbon: we need to have both together – and lower embodied carbon too!

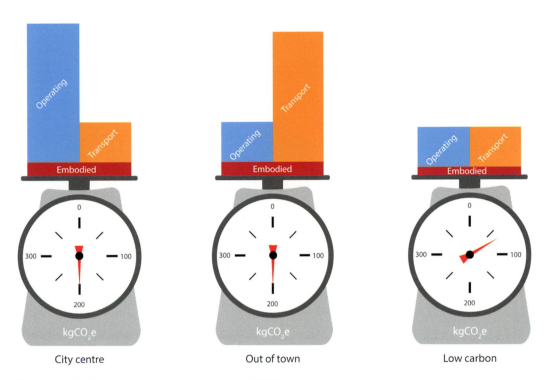

Fig 5.4 Tipping the scales towards low carbon buildings

In this chapter, an indicative whole carbon benchmark of around 200 kgCO$_2$e/m^2 of GIA per annum has been suggested as typical for a UK office building based on a 60-year assessment period. However, it is rather pointless to establish a benchmark if it doesn't then stimulate any further action. Now that the whole carbon footprint has been, somewhat crudely, defined, the next step is to do something to reduce it.

Part 2 of this book provides some practical guidance on how to reduce operating, embodied and transport energy and CO$_2$e emissions during the design, construction and operation of buildings.

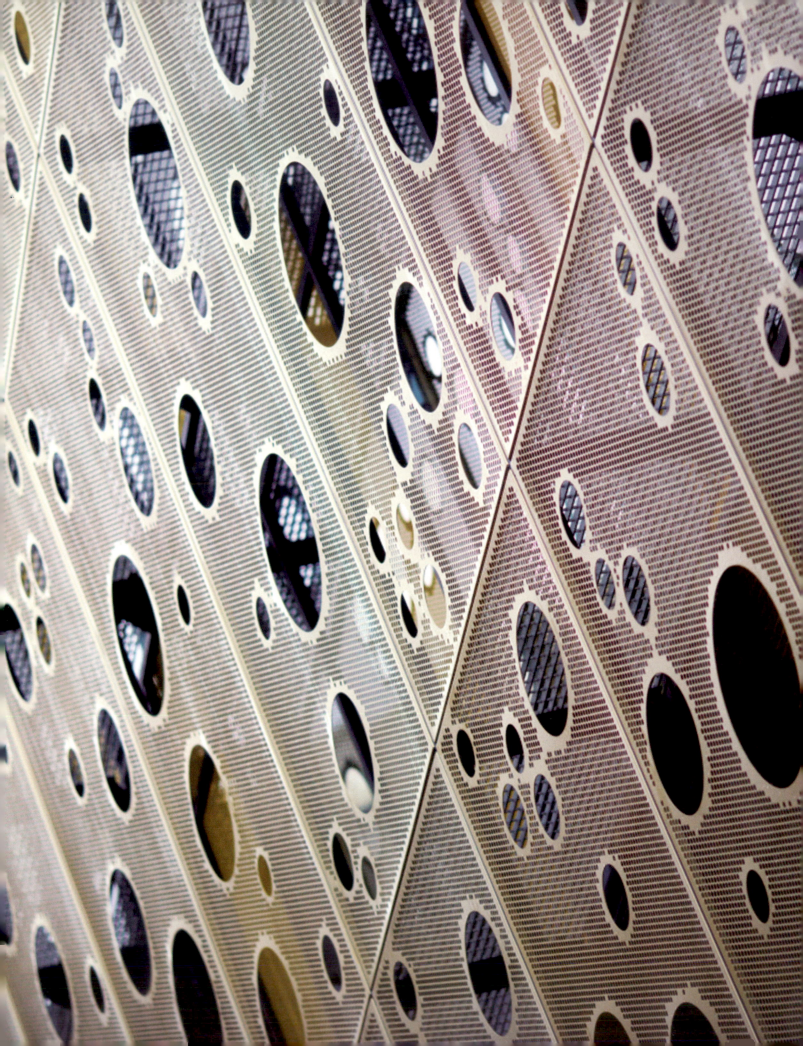

Part 2

CHANGING COLOUR
Reducing energy and carbon in buildings

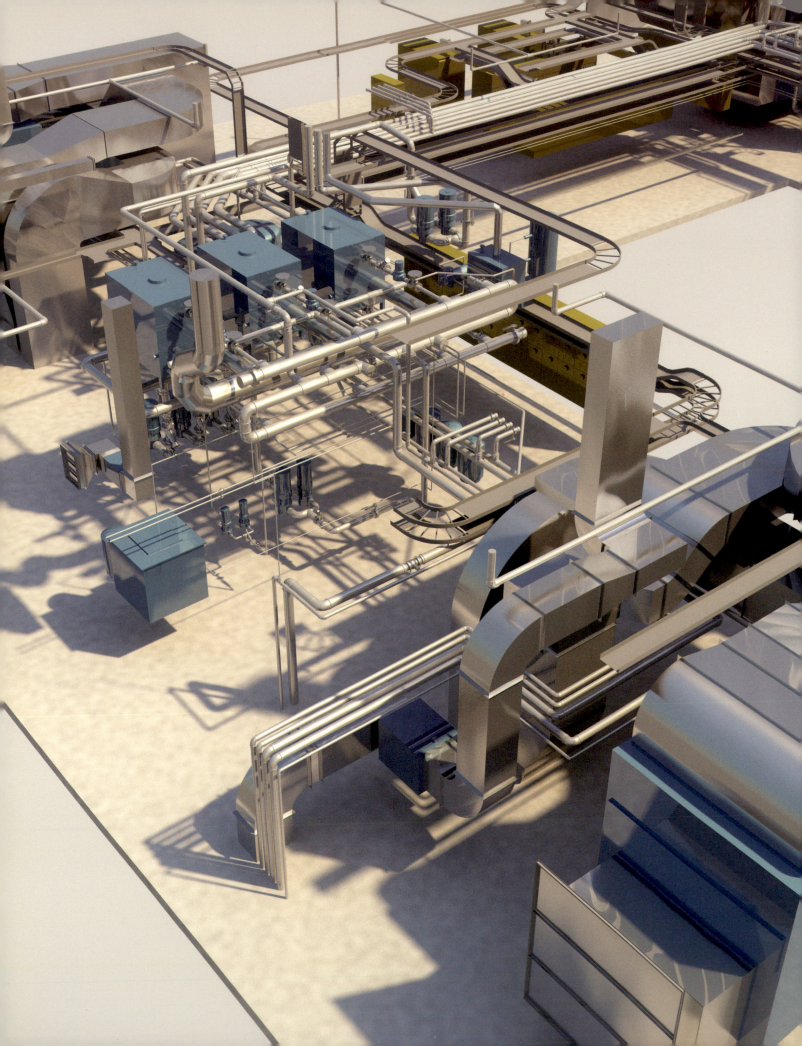

Chapter 6

Ten steps to reducing energy consumption

Normal people ... believe that if it ain't broke, don't fix it. Engineers believe that if it ain't broke, it doesn't have enough features yet.

Scott Adams,
The Dilbert Principle, Boxtree Limited, 1997

The ten steps to reducing energy consumption set out in this chapter can be applied to the design of new buildings and the refurbishment and operation of existing buildings. The first issues are to identify the extent of consumption and where and when it is being used (step 1) and to challenge standard design assumptions related to lighting and comfort (step 2). Next, consider the building fabric (step 3), which does not consume energy directly, but does influence consumption due to ventilation (step 4), heating and cooling (step 5) and lighting (step 6). The equipment plugged in by the occupants (step 7) and miscellaneous other services, such as domestic hot water and lifts (step 8), complete the energy-consuming items in the building. The building may work brilliantly on paper, but if the systems are not set up correctly, handed over with clear instructions and then carefully maintained (step 9), then they will not work efficiently.

Finally, the influence of people must be considered. Empty buildings do not use much energy. It is the people in buildings that lead to energy use, so it is important to engage with the occupants and make it easy for them to save energy (step 10).

6.1 UNDERSTANDING WHERE ENERGY IS USED

The first step to reducing the operating carbon footprint of a building is to understand how the energy is being used. This may sound obvious, but many buildings were, or are, designed to (just) pass the building regulations current at the time of construction, with no serious consideration given to reducing actual operating energy consumption. This is particularly prevalent in speculative/commercial offices – the developer or building owner does not pay the energy bills and so lowest capital cost is often the primary investment criteria. Chapter 10 discusses the business case for investment in energy reduction and low carbon buildings.

Figure 6.1 shows the breakdown of operating carbon for an air conditioned office building based on the typical and best practice benchmarks in ECON 19 (excluding humidification) and the Target Emission Rate (TER) for a typical Building Regulations 2010 Part L compliant building (which is also used in the calculation of the Energy Performance Certificate (EPC) rating).[1]

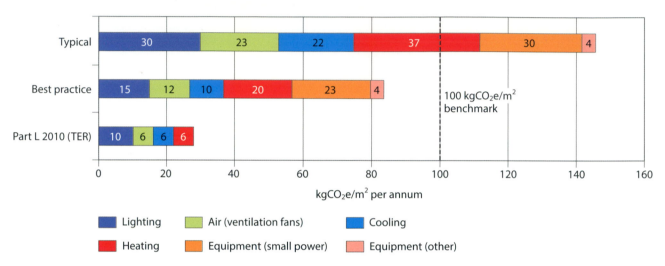

Fig 6.1 Breakdown of energy consumption in typical air conditioned office based on Type 3 ECON 19 benchmarks and Building Regulations 2010 Part L energy modelling

As discussed in Chapter 2, an office building can appear very efficient in the computer model, but have actual energy consumption over five times greater than the EPC and Part L modelling output. This is because the modelling is a measure of the energy efficiency of the façade and the services for regulatory compliance purposes only. It does not assess whether the design is appropriate (i.e. is the design efficient or oversized?) and does not attempt to estimate annual energy consumption. Unfortunately, this subtlety is not widely appreciated.

In Chapter 2, energy consumption in office buildings was identified as being due to LEACHs. To assist in identifying the impact of these on the operating carbon of buildings, the breakdown in Table 6.1 can be considered as a very rough guide.

From 2018, all existing commercial office buildings in the UK will require a minimum E-rated EPC before they can be leased or sold.[2] The easiest way to achieve this will be by improving the lighting, as this typically accounts for 35% of the EPC rating. While this is a positive step forward, the focus of legislation really needs to be on reducing the actual energy consumption of buildings and not just the energy efficiency of their components.

	Typical energy-consuming items	Typical % of kgCO$_2$e
Lighting	Internal and external lights	20%
Equipment	Computers, printers, fridges, lifts, security systems, servers and other plug-in equipment/appliances	30%
Air	Fans (supply and exhaust)	15%
Cooling	Chillers and pumps	15%
Heating	Space heating boiler, domestic hot water boiler and pumps	20%

Table 6.1 Typical operating carbon breakdown for UK office buildings

Figure 6.2 (overleaf) shows the components which influence the actual energy consumption in office buildings, and those which are typically addressed in building regulations (regulated energy). The numbers in brackets show the other 9 steps which are discussed in the remaining sections in this chapter.

During the design stage, two energy models should really be used – one to calculate the regulated energy (building regulations and EPC) and one to estimate the actual energy consumption (i.e. the total annual energy bills). The latter should include a sensitivity analysis of assumptions made – a good example is the NABERS energy modelling protocol in Australia.[3]

In existing buildings the key requirement is to understand how the energy is actually being used. Many buildings only have a single meter for each utility (electricity and gas) which makes it difficult to identify and target specific items to reduce energy. Under UK building regulations new commercial buildings are required to install meters and sub-meters so that 90% of the energy consumption of each fuel can be assigned to various end uses (such as heating and lighting).[4] In buildings greater than 1,000 m^2 an automatic meter data collection system is also required. Unfortunately, most existing commercial office buildings do not have such metering arrangements. Installing permanent or temporary sub-meters to key systems can greatly assist in identifying and then verifying energy reduction measures.

A large amount of energy is wasted by systems which are not turned off when they should be. Good metering can help to identify this. However, too much metering can lead to data overload. Numerous software tools are now available to analyse the data and display it in meaningful ways, and provide the ability to drill down into the detail when necessary to investigate potential issues. Appendix H provides more guidance on metering and energy management plans.

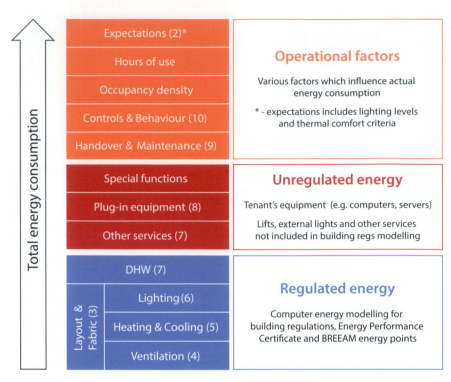

Fig 6.2 Typical energy consumption components – regulated, unregulated and operating

PLANNING FOR LOW CARBON BUILDINGS

In 2010, a 1960s office building in the centre of Manchester had an operating energy consumption of 255 $kgCO_2e/m^2$ (the suggested benchmark in Chapter 2 is 100 $kgCO_2e/m^2$). The 900 m^2 building has a single constant air volume air handling unit (AHU) supplying air to four floors. A chiller provides chilled water to a cooling coil in the AHU. A gas boiler provides heating hot water to the AHU and heater batteries in the air supply to each floor. The tenants have their own utility electricity meters for small power and lighting.

The landlord electricity supply has a half-hourly meter which, since 2010, was tracked through a web-based energy monitoring system. This plots the half-hourly data on monthly charts. After reviewing the charts, the landlord realised that the AHU was operating 24/7 and took steps to reduce its running hours. The timer clock was reset to turn the system off during the evenings (6 p.m. to 7.15 a.m.) and all weekend. This represents a 67% reduction in hours of operation, and resulted in a 60% reduction in landlord electricity consumption. Changing the AHU timer clock also resulted in a net reduction in gas consumption.[5] The total energy consumtion of the building was reduced to 140 $kgCO_2e/m^2$ for no capital cost.

The effect of turning the AHU system off can be seen graphically in the profile of the half-hourly meter electricity charts in Figure 6.3, which were produced by a web-based energy monitoring system.

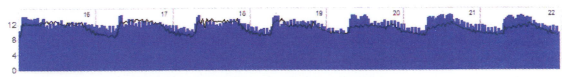

16 – 22 May 2011 – almost constant electricity consumption at night and weekends

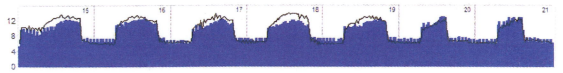

15 – 21 Aug 2011 – consumption at night reduced but system still running at weekend

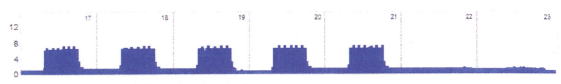

17 – 23 Oct 2011 – AHU turned off at night and weekends

Fig 6.3 Half-hourly meter readings of landlord electricity for three different weeks in a Manchester office building

This example illustrates how, for no cost, major reductions in energy consumption can be made, simply by using the off switch. How many other buildings have systems running when no one is in them? Without adequate metering it is often not obvious that systems are still running at 2 a.m. on Sundays. The AHU timer was not the only energy issue in the building and cost effective measures have been identified which could reduce the energy consumption to 80 to 90 $kgCO_2e/m^2$, primarily by improving lighting and controls. Getting energy consumption under 100 $kgCO_2e/m^2$ is possible in many office buildings.

6.2 WHATEVER YOU WANT: CHALLENGING THE STATUS QUO

If I had asked my customers what they wanted, they would have told me a faster horse.

Attributed to Henry Ford

The default for office design in the UK over the past 20 years has been to set the air conditioning to 22 °C all year round and provide 500 lux lighting[6] across the whole floor plate. This leads to sealed air conditioned boxes with excessive lighting, which in turn results in unnecessary capital cost and higher energy consumption.

Unfortunately, this standard is now so ingrained that many developers or designers don't stop to think if there is another way of delivering a comfortable, functional building. Or, if they do, the investors or tenant's agents pull out a standard industry checklist that has 22 °C and 500 lux on it, and so the developer/designer delivers the building to 'respond to market demands'. The sustainability box is ticked by obtaining a design energy rating (EPC) and a BREEAM certificate, both of which can be easily achieved by providing energy efficient services rather than low energy buildings.

To break away from standard design requires selling the benefits of alternative approaches to investors, owners, agents and tenants. This is a major challenge.

Lighting levels

The primary purpose of lighting in office buildings is to ensure that building occupants have enough light to perform their tasks well and without excessive eye strain. Good lighting, both daylighting and artificial, combined with views to the outside, can help to avoid errors, prevent premature fatigue and improve productivity.[7] Daylight and views are discussed in the next section on façades.

In most offices the tasks to be performed are either paper- or screen-based, and confined to a relatively small area of a desk or workstation. There are two methods of delivering the minimum lighting levels at a workstation, as shown in Figure 6.4:

- **Blanket**: provide lighting across the whole floor plate so that the minimum lighting level is achieved at any conceivable desk location both now and in the future.
- **Task**: provide lighting only at the locations it is needed, by positioning ceiling lights over desks or using desk lamps (with ceiling lights providing background lighting).

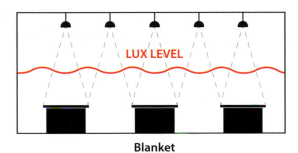
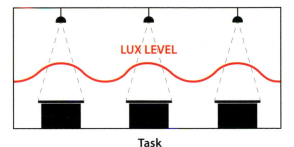

Fig 6.4 Blanket v task lighting approaches

Most offices adopt the blanket lighting approach. Table 6.2 shows the typical installed lighting power density (W/m² of NLA) and the annual energy consumption and cost based on:

- the lighting being on for 2,600 hours per year
- efficient T5 fluorescent ceiling lighting
- 6 W task lamps with one workstation per 12 m² of NLA (= 0.5 W/m²)
- an electricity tariff of 10p/kWh.

	Method of lighting	Workstation lux level	Background lux level	W/m²	kWh/m²	Cost per 1,000 m²
1	Blanket	500	500	12	31	£3,100
2	Blanket	300	300	8	21	£2,100
3	Task	300	200	5	13	£1,300
4	Task	300	50	2	5	£500

Table 6.2 Indicative lighting power density and energy consumption for different lighting approaches

If a task-based lighting approach is adopted then significant savings in lighting energy consumption can be made. This requires coordination and agreement between the landlord and tenant, particularly in speculative offices where the tendency is to install all the lighting first, and bring in the tenant afterwards. This approach can result in the tenant then ripping out the newly installed lighting (sending it all to waste) and installing their own. Shell and core delivery methods, where the floor covering, ceiling and building services are not installed in the tenant's area until it is let, should therefore be encouraged in speculative buildings.

ENERGY EFFICIENCY VERSUS EFFICIENT DESIGN

To illustrate the difference between energy efficiency and efficient design, consider the two options for lighting in a meeting room as shown in Table 6.3. Both options have the same light fittings (lumens per Watt) and so are treated as having the same energy efficiency by Part L and EPC ratings. But the room with three fittings will have half the annual energy consumption. Designing for low energy is a function of both quality (efficiency) and quantity (total power installed and hours of operation). This is one reason (of many) for the performance gap between design energy ratings and metered energy consumption.

Number of fittings	3	6
Lux level on working plane	400 lux	660 lux
Efficiency	56 lumens/Watt	56 lumens/Watt
Total power	190 W	380 W
kWh/year (5 hours × 240 days)	228 kWh	456 kWh

Table 6.3 **Lighting options for a meeting room to show efficiency v consumption**

Thermal comfort

Thermal comfort is not measured by air temperature but by the number of occupants not complaining. It is defined in ISO 7730:2005 as: 'that condition of mind which expresses satisfaction with the thermal environment'.

Thermal comfort is therefore very subjective and an individual's perception of whether they are too hot or too cold varies considerably, often between two people sitting next to each other in the same office. It is not unusual to find an electric heater plugged in under someone's desk, even if the rest of the occupants feel warm. The adage 'you can't please all of the people all of the time' is particularly applicable to thermal comfort. A total of 80% of occupants is the usual target for the minimum number of people who should be thermally comfortable in an office environment.[8] This still means that one in five will be dissatisfied!

An individual's perception of thermal comfort is influenced by six physical factors: air temperature, humidity, radiant temperature, air movement, clothing and their level of activity. Psychological factors also have an influence – for example, people will often tolerate wider temperature ranges if they feel they have some degree of control over their environment. People living in tropical countries will generally have a higher tolerance of hot, humid conditions than those living somewhere cold like Scotland. We adapt to the climate and modify our behaviour, clothing and expectations to suit – or, as we are discussing thermal comfort in offices, perhaps it should be 'to not to suit'.

A building's façade, internal thermal mass, and heating, air conditioning and ventilation (HVAC) systems will influence four of the physical factors: indoor air temperature, relative humidity, mean radiant temperature and air movement. However, the comfort criteria for office buildings is usually only defined in design briefs using air temperature and humidity. Table 6.4 shows typical air temperature criteria for UK offices.[9]

Building type	Summer	Winter
Air conditioned	24 °C +/-2 °C	20 °C +/- 2 °C
Mixed mode/naturally ventilated	To not exceed 25 °C for 5%, and 28 °C for 1%, of occupied hours	

Table 6.4 **Typical air temperature design criteria for offices in the UK (British Council for Offices, 2009)**

Figure 6.5 (overleaf) shows the limitation of using only air temperature to define thermal comfort by illustrating how a person's perception of comfort changes in summer with changes in other physical factors – whether they are sitting or active, in sun or shade, wearing light or warm clothing or have air movement over their skin – even if the air temperature and humidity remain constant. In winter the direction of the thermal comfort arrow is reversed.

Since activity and air speed in mechanically ventilated office buildings are assumed to be reasonably consistent all year round, the operative temperature[10] – a combination of air temperature and radiant temperature – can be used to better reflect comfort than air temperature alone. The typical ranges stated in CIBSE Guide A (Table 1.5) are 21 to 23 °C for winter and 22 to 24 °C for summer. These are quite narrow bands. The BCO *Guide to Specification 2009* recommends a limit of 26 to 27 °C.

People adapt to the changing seasons outside work, usually dressing differently in summer than in winter, but then turn up at work in the same uniform all year

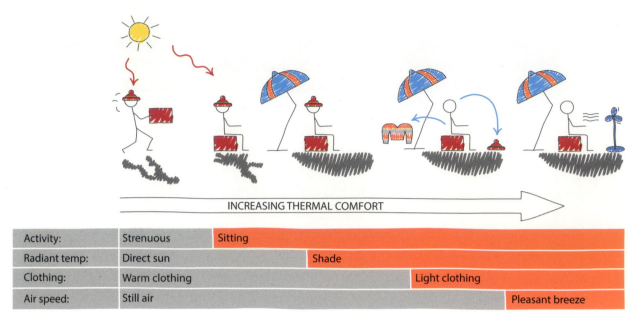

Activity:	Strenuous	Sitting		
Radiant temp:	Direct sun		Shade	
Clothing:	Warm clothing			Light clothing
Air speed:	Still air				Pleasant breeze

Fig 6.5 **Changing perceptions of thermal comfort while air temperature and humidity remain constant**

round. Changing clothing seasonally is an obvious solution, but does require a cultural shift from employers and employees – from suits to smart casual. The Japanese have been promoting this for some time through the Cool Biz initiative.[11]

Adopting an adaptive approach to thermal comfort,[12] and widening the temperature range in a building, will save heating and cooling energy, although the impact on productivity also needs to be considered.[13] An adaptive approach reduces the thermostat set point to suit the external conditions. This can be done through a floating set point linked to external temperature sensors, although a simpler solution is to just change the set point every 3 months. A potential strategy is shown in Table 6.5. To implement seasonal temperature bands, without incurring a barrage of complaints, requires a clear communication strategy with occupants – refer to Appendix H for further details.

	Heating	Cooling	Single system
Winter	20 °C	Off	20 °C
Spring	20 °C	24 °C	22 °C
Summer	Off	26 °C	26 °C
Autumn	20 °C	24 °C	22 °C

Table 6.5 **Potential seasonal set point strategy**

To improve people's perception of thermal comfort in office buildings the following initiatives can also be considered:

- provide individual control of thermal environment (e.g. opening windows, use of blinds)
- allow people to move out of sunny areas
- provide flexible working hours so people can work at more comfortable times (e.g. allowing siestas in hot climates)
- provide cold drinks in summer
- increase air movement in summer using local desk or ceiling fans (the cooling effect can be equivalent to reducing the operative temperature by around 2 °C).

The biggest challenge with office buildings is convincing occupants (and the tenant's representatives) that they can be comfortable without mechanical cooling to 22 °C. The main barrier to adopting adaptive thermal comfort criteria is all in the mind.

THEORY VERSUS PRACTICE

The Cundall Manchester office is on the tenth floor of a typical 1960s office building in the centre of the city next to a coach station and a very busy bus route. The windows face south-east and north-west. The ceiling height is 2.6 m, the floor plate depth is 16 m and there is little thermal mass. The landlord has a detailed report from a highly regarded international engineering practice that natural ventilation doesn't really work and that the best solution for energy and comfort is to replace the whole façade (20 storeys), seal the building and install mechanical ventilation.

This recommendation represents a significant capital cost to the landlord. It also ignores the fact that the building works fairly well without comfort cooling most of the year. On a 26 °C day the high-level operable windows (which are equivalent to only 2% of the floor area) are all open and the office is reasonably comfortable. The cooling system hasn't been switched on for over a year. It may not work in engineering theory, but it seems to work fine in practice. If we couldn't open the windows Cundall would move out of the building.

6.3 BUILDING FABRIC

The building fabric (façade and roof) forms an interface between the inside and outside. The façade is the most visible component of a building, and a great deal of attention is usually spent on how it looks, either to blend in or to make a statement. Until the introduction of more stringent Building Regulations few façades were designed or constructed with energy efficiency in mind. Most are still now only designed to just pass the minimum legislative requirements.

The façade influences many aspects of a building's performance and the experience of occupants. Since we spend most (up to 90%) of our lives inside buildings,[14] it is important to design façades from the inside out, and not just from the outside in. Figure 6.6 illustrates some of the factors to consider when designing a new façade, or improving an existing one.

The factors that directly influence energy use are described in more detail in Appendix H and include:

- daylight – on working surfaces allowing lights to be turned off
- glare – pulling blinds down reduces daylight
- solar gain – raises air and radiant temperatures, increasing demand for cooling
- cold surfaces – create discomfort in winter, increasing demand for heating
- insulation and thermal bridging – heat losses and gains through conduction
- air tightness – heat losses and gains through convection
- openings – is natural ventilation provided to avoid/reduce fan energy consumption?
- noise and pollution – these factors can prevent the use of openings for ventilation.

A façade comprises a kit of parts which can be put together to give the optimum solution in a particular climate. These parts include:

- proportion of glazing to solid elements
- type of glass – U-value, solar heat gain coefficient (SHGC or g-value), visible light transmission (t-value) and reflectivity
- type of framing system – U-value, thermal bridging, air permeability
- type of solid wall – U-value, thermal bridging, air permeability
- type of shading – fixed or operable
- type of blinds – rollers or venetians, manual or automated[15]
- ventilation openings – manual or automated, louvres or windows.

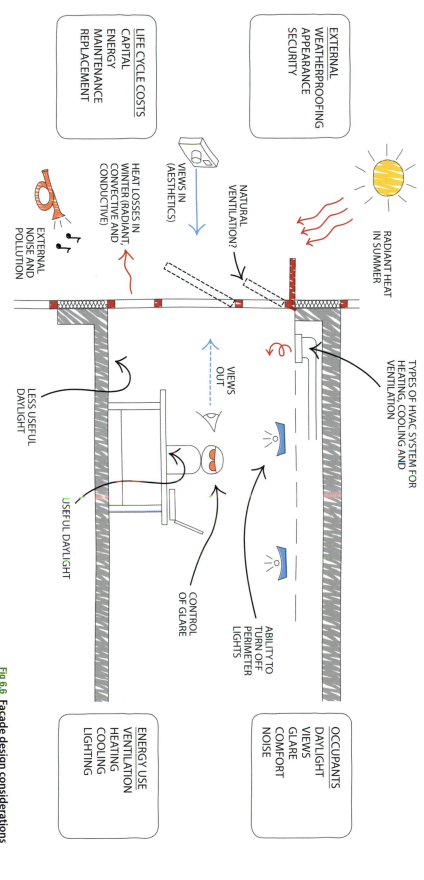

EXTERNAL
WEATHERPROOFING
APPEARANCE
SECURITY

LIFE CYCLE COSTS
CAPITAL
ENERGY
MAINTENANCE
REPLACEMENT

VIEWS IN
(AESTHETICS)

HEAT LOSSES IN
WINTER (RADIANT,
CONVECTIVE AND
CONDUCTIVE)

NATURAL
VENTILATION?

EXTERNAL
NOISE AND
POLLUTION

RADIANT HEAT
IN SUMMER

TYPES OF HVAC SYSTEM FOR
HEATING, COOLING AND
VENTILATION

LESS USEFUL
DAYLIGHT

VIEWS
OUT

USEFUL DAYLIGHT

CONTROL
OF GLARE

ABILITY TO
TURN OFF
PERIMETER
LIGHTS

OCCUPANTS
DAYLIGHT
VIEWS
GLARE
COMFORT
NOISE

ENERGY USE
VENTILATION
HEATING
COOLING
LIGHTING

Fig 6.6 Façade design considerations

East- and west-facing glass is harder to shade effectively than north- and south-facing glass. So, does every face of the building have to look the same, or should each respond to its solar orientation? If the façade must look the same on every face then it will invariably compromise optimum energy and comfort performance because the sun doesn't stay still and affects each façade differently.

The art in designing a good façade lies in addressing the above issues, while also considering capital cost, maintenance, cleaning, security and, of course, aesthetics. Given the number of variables, the design of a high performance façade, appropriate to the building form and location, is limited only by the imagination, skill and integration of the project team – architect, engineer, acoustician, lighting designer, suppliers, contractor and cost consultant.

To illustrate the interaction between daylight, energy and thermal comfort of different façade designs, an analysis of nine options is summarised in Appendix H. These include full height glazing, vertical panels, horizontal strips and punched windows with a range of external shading and internal blinds. Each option is assessed for north, south, east and west orientations for a building in London.

In existing buildings there is often less scope for creativity, particularly if the building has a listed façade. Half of the office stock in England and Wales was built before 1970, with one-quarter before 1940[16] which is before building regulations requiring good thermal performance were in place.[17]

Thermographic imaging and air tightness testing can be used to quantify the performance of existing façades (and new ones), although in most existing buildings it is usually obvious where the problems lie – a visual inspection and discussions with building occupants on the subjects of glare, solar gain and draughts will quickly identify these.

EXISTING FAÇADES: FIVE QUICK WAYS TO REDUCE ENERGY (AND IMPROVE COMFORT)

1 Seal up gaps and cracks, particularly at wall, floor and window interfaces.
2 Install a solar film on clear glass – but select carefully to avoid making spaces too dark.
3 Install better blinds which have reflective (and potentially thermal) properties.
4 If possible, give occupants the ability to open windows (provided that air conditioning can be turned off locally).
5 Fit cavity wall insulation or insulated plasterboard (but check implications of condensation on the cold surface interface with the insulation).

Ultimately, there is no idealised façade design and most façades will have to balance a variety of competing requirements including:

- letting light in – but limiting solar gain in the summer
- providing views out – but avoiding glare
- letting air in (where and when required) – but keeping out noise, dust, insects and unwanted people
- high performance – but still affordable.

6.4 VENTILATION

Fresh air is required in buildings to limit CO_2 concentrations and to provide acceptable indoor air quality (reducing odours and indoor pollutants). Ventilation, which can include recirculated air, is required to deliver fresh air, and can also be used to control moisture (to reduce the risk of condensation and mould growth) and remove excess heat (for thermal comfort). There are three standard methods of ventilating a building:

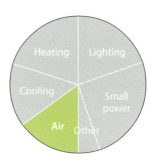

- natural – typically by openable windows/louvres
- mechanical – fans and ducts
- mixed mode – a combination of natural and mechanical methods.

Before the widespread adoption of air conditioning systems, buildings were naturally ventilated and the vernacular architecture reflects this. Over the past 40 years the majority of speculative office buildings in the UK have been mechanically ventilated without openable windows. Natural ventilation tends to be limited to smaller office developments. The reasons for using mechanical ventilation include:

- narrow internal air temperature bands specified
- requirements to keep out external noise, reduce ingress of external contaminants (including dust, insects and exhaust fumes) and provide better security
- the floor plates are too deep (greater than 15 m) for natural ventilation to work effectively
- the façades have too much glass and air conditioning is required to remove the heat due to solar gain
- market demand – the perception of tenants that an air-conditioned office is a higher quality building.

So prevalent is the glass-clad air conditioned office block that some designers may go through their entire career without having to design a naturally ventilated building. It is much easier to design a sealed box and pump air around it than to work out natural air flows, the types of window/louvre openings and who controls them. Unfortunately, the electricity consumption of the fans and cooling systems resulting from the mechanical approach can account for around one-third of an office building's operating carbon.[18]

The need to build low energy buildings will see an increase in mixed mode offices. These use natural ventilation when no heating or cooling is required (with wider temperature bands to extend the hours during which this occurs) and efficient mechanical ventilation (with heat recovery) when in heating and/or cooling mode. As shown in Figures 2.5, 2.7 and 2.8 in Chapter 2, the office buildings with the lowest operating carbon tend to be those with the ability to open windows.

As mixed mode buildings are perceived to have higher capital costs, having both openable windows/louvres and mechanical ventilation, they are typically built by owner-occupiers who see the benefit of lower energy bills and increased resilience. However, this trend is changing and some commercial office developers are starting to offer mixed mode offices to the UK market.

FRESH AIR REQUIREMENTS IN OFFICE BUILDINGS

'Fresh air' is air brought inside the building from the outside, by natural or mechanical means. It is also known as 'outside air' as some engineers question whether polluted air outside can be considered to be fresh. In this book the term 'fresh air' is generally used on the basis that we don't say, 'I just need a good breath of outside air'.

There is no universally agreed minimum volume of fresh air to be provided in office buildings, although values of 8 to 10 litres of air per second per person (l/s/person) are typically used.[19] To improve the indoor air quality in buildings, the minimum fresh air can be increased but this results in increased energy consumption due to the need for larger fans (to move the air around) and heating and cooling larger quantities of fresh air. In the UK, the BREEAM rating tool does not provide points for increasing the fresh air quantities. In the USA and Australia, the LEED and Green Star rating tools both award points for higher volumes of fresh air and consequently more offices are designed with fresh air rates greater than 10 l/s/person.[20]

The fresh air requirements for naturally ventilated buildings are not usually expressed in l/s/person as it is not possible to provide fresh air naturally at a constant rate. The approach typically used is to limit the average CO_2 concentrations during the day to be equivalent to the air quality provided by 10 l/s/person of mechanical ventilation. As a rule of thumb, a minimum free ventilation area (through windows, louvres, etc.), expressed as a percentage of the floor area served, of around 5% is typically assumed for naturally ventilated systems to provide fresh air and remove heat in the UK.[21]

Making natural ventilation work

The carbon benefit of natural ventilation is based on the assumption that providing occupants with tolerable conditions, and the means to change them, uses less energy (no fans or cooling) than providing better conditions but with limited or no means of individual control. Occupants can make their own decisions on how to balance the often competing requirements between ventilation rate, external noise, draughts and views out (blinds up or down).

Natural ventilation makes use of wind forces (wind effect) and differences in air temperature (stack effect) to move air through a building. The most common methods, with some simple rules of thumb, are shown in Figure 6.7.

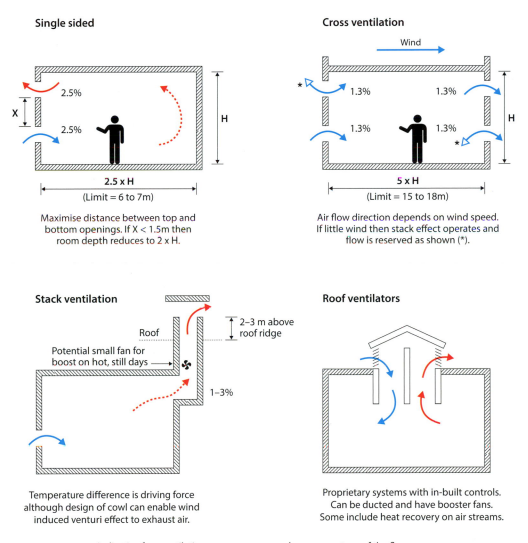

Single sided

2.5%

X

2.5%

H

2.5 x H
(Limit = 6 to 7m)

Maximise distance between top and bottom openings. If X < 1.5m then room depth reduces to 2 x H.

Cross ventilation

Wind

* 1.3%   1.3%

1.3%   1.3%

*

H

5 x H
(Limit = 15 to 18m)

Air flow direction depends on wind speed. If little wind then stack effect operates and flow is reserved as shown (*).

Stack ventilation

2–3 m above roof ridge

Roof

Potential small fan for boost on hot, still days

1–3%

Temperature difference is driving force although design of cowl can enable wind induced venturi effect to exhaust air.

Roof ventilators

Proprietary systems with in-built controls. Can be ducted and have booster fans. Some include heat recovery on air streams.

Indicative free ventilation areas are expressed as a percentage of the floor area

Fig 6.7 Typical types of natural ventilation

Of these natural ventilation methods, the most commonly used in office buildings are single sided and cross ventilation. The design and analysis of natural ventilation can become quite complex, particularly when the rules of thumb are exceeded or when the total internal cooling load, including solar gain, exceeds 40 W/m². If the internal occupancy is more than one person per 10 m² then internal heat gain due to lights, equipment and people alone could exceed this value.[22] However, unlike designing mechanical systems, natural ventilation should be based on average gains over the day rather than peak conditions. This takes into account the fact that the lights may be off when the sun is shining, some equipment will be in standby and the actual occupancy is probably less than the total number of seats.

The majority of software and design tools available to mechanical engineers are for sealed buildings with air conditioning, where conditions are relatively stable. Natural ventilation is highly variable because, at any given moment, both the rate of ventilation and the pattern of air flow are affected by the prevailing weather conditions – differences in air temperatures, wind speed and wind direction. When other potential issues, including dust, noise, security, thermal mass and control, are added to the design challenges, it is understandable that developers, designers and tenants invariably go for sealed buildings with air conditioning – they are simpler to design, easier to control and carry less risk.

One, often overlooked, advantage of natural ventilation is that it works even when the power is off. On a hot day, any power failure will rapidly make a sealed glass air conditioned building uninhabitable.

If you do have a naturally ventilated building, or are contemplating designing one, then Appendix H provides some guidance on how to improve the effectiveness of the ventilation. If natural ventilation cannot work, or is not an acceptable solution, then a mechanical ventilation system will be required.

Reducing the energy consumption of mechanical ventilation

Most mechanical systems use fans and ducts to supply and exhaust air to and from individual spaces in buildings. Figure 6.8 shows the typical arrangement for a supply and exhaust ventilation system air handling unit (AHU).

The volume of air required to remove heat from a space is based on the cooling mechanism used. If heat is removed by extracting hot air (e.g. air-based cooling systems) then the supply air volume required will depend, among other things, on the supply air temperature and the desired internal air temperature. A similar mechanism applies when supply air is used for heating a space. In both cases, the total volume of supply air needed for heating/cooling does not have to comprise 100% fresh

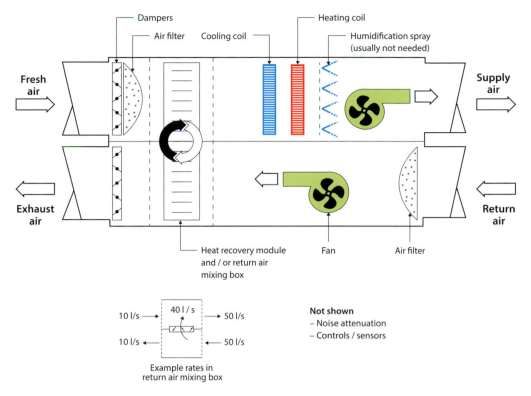

10 l/s → | 40 l/s | → 50 l/s
10 l/s ← | | ← 50 l/s

Example rates in
return air mixing box

Not shown
– Noise attenuation
– Controls / sensors

Fig 6.8 **Typical components of an air handling unit**

air and most HVAC systems are designed to recirculate return air and mix in the minimum fresh air requirement (typically 8 to 10 l/s/person).

If heating (e.g. radiators) or cooling (e.g. chilled beams) occurs directly in the space then the supply air ventilation rate is usually based on the fresh air requirement only. This reduces the size of fans and ducts required, which is why chilled beam systems usually use less energy than air-based cooling systems – water is much more efficient at transporting heat energy than air. The types of heating and cooling systems are discussed in Section 6.5.

The operating carbon associated with mechanical ventilation is due to fan energy consumption. The energy to heat and cool the supply air is discussed in Section 6.5. The energy efficiency of the ventilation system, measured in specific fan power (watts per l/s), is influenced by:

- the efficiency of the fan/motor:
    - type of motor
    - efficiency at normal operation, not just peak capacity
- the resistance to air flow in the air distribution system:
    - size and shape of ducts – smaller/flatter ducts have increased air resistance
    - restrictions to air flow (filters, bends, dirt, etc.)
- how the system is controlled.

The most efficient fans have an efficiency of between 60 and 80% depending on their size and configuration. However, in most existing buildings, the fans are likely to operate at half this efficiency.[23]

In variable air flow systems, fans should be selected to operate at their best efficiency for the typical, not peak, air flow rates. When fans operate at less than 30 to 40% capacity their energy efficiency drops off significantly. Avoiding the use of oversized fans will allow them to operate in their most efficient range for longer periods. A well-designed air distribution system (fans and ducts) should have a specific fan power of less than 2 W per l/s, with very efficient systems close to 1 W per l/s.

Whether the building has the most efficient ventilation system, or has an old system with poor performance, one of the easiest ways of saving energy is to turn it off when it is not needed. Lighting, despite being highly visible, is often left on overnight, so it is perhaps not surprising that fans, which are hidden from view, are often left running all night. A 1 kW fan left running 24/7 (8,760 hours/annum) will cost £900 to run and will release 5 tCO_2e in a year.

Appendix H provides further guidance on reducing the energy consumption of mechanical ventilation systems.

INCREASING FRESH AIR: THERMAL VERSUS FAN ENERGY

If higher than minimum fresh air volumes are provided then this increases the energy required to heat and cool the air. This is a key tension in green buildings – improve the indoor air quality but also increase the energy consumption. The use of heat recovery systems to preheat/cool the outside air by transferring heat from/to the return air can help, but this introduces air resistance which increases fan energy consumption. When the heat recovery potential is small, the heat recovery system should be bypassed to reduce this. The systems should ideally be able to recover both sensible (dry) and latent (wet) heat.

Mixed mode systems

Mixed mode is basically a combination of the two systems, either with fans working alongside natural ventilation to boost air flows (supply or exhaust) or as two separate systems with the building operating in either natural or mechanical mode only, depending on the climate conditions and ventilation requirements at a given point in time. The Passivhaus[24] methodology is an example of a separate mixed mode approach:

- mechanical ventilation and heat recovery in the winter to minimise heat losses due to supplying fresh air
- natural ventilation in summer via openable windows.

Figure 6.9 shows an example mixed mode strategy in an office compared to natural ventilation and full air conditioning (HVAC).

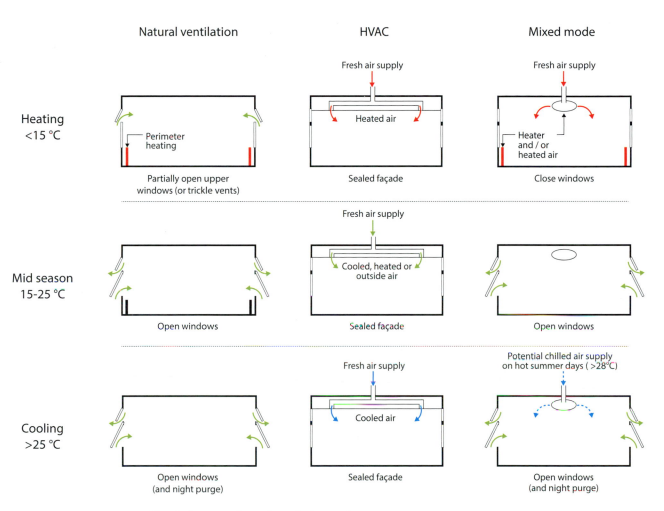

Fig 6.9 **Simplistic comparison of ventilation modes**

For mixed mode buildings to be successful an appropriate control strategy must be developed, and the building occupants must engage with this. Making it fully automatic is often not successful – natural ventilation relies on giving people a degree of control. If you take this away then it may not be too long before the openable windows are permanently closed and the building runs in mechanical mode only.

Another key challenge with a mixed mode approach in offices is the cost of installing both a mechanical and a naturally ventilated system. Façades without openable windows are cheaper than those with, and consequently it is often difficult to justify mixed mode on an energy cost saving basis alone. However, to future-proof buildings to provide flexibility, business continuity during power shortages and reduced exposure to rising energy prices and carbon taxes, constructing buildings with the ability to open windows whenever possible makes a lot of sense – although it might require legislation to make this happen.[25]

6.5 HEATING AND COOLING

Heating and cooling typically accounts for one-third of a commercial office building's operating carbon foot-print in the UK[26] and is influenced by a number of factors including:

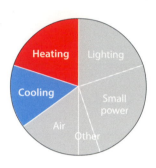

- climate
- internal temperatures to be achieved (Section 6.2)
- thermal performance of the façade (Section 6.3)
- fresh air supplied to occupants (Section 6.4)
- efficiency of the heating and cooling system
- hours of operation.

A building with a good façade and high internal loads (people, lights and equipment) will still usually require some heating in the winter, primarily of the fresh air supplied to the occupants. Unless a building relies solely on natural ventilation, some form of cooling is provided in most modern office buildings. Any system which provides cooling is commonly referred to as air conditioning, although the correct terms are:

- comfort cooling – controls air temperature only
- air conditioning – controls both air temperature and humidity.

There are many systems for heating and cooling office buildings which use different methods of generating, distributing and then transferring thermal energy to provide the occupants with thermal comfort. The three most common methods of providing heating and cooling energy are:

- hot and/or chilled water supplied from central plant (refer to Figure 6.10)
- F-gases (refrigerant) supplied by heat pumps, either central or distributed
- direct gas or electric heating in the space.

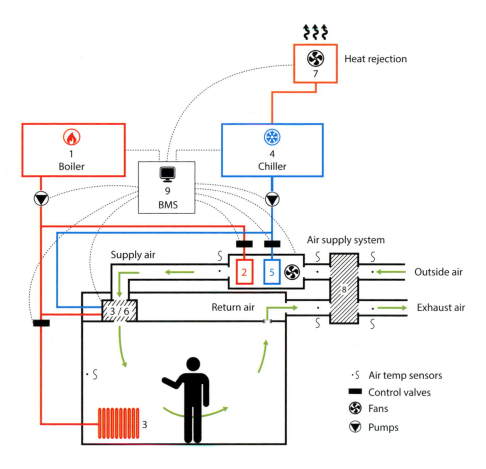

Heat rejection

1. Heat source – typically a gas boiler
2. Heating coils in AHU
3. Heat emitter in space (e.g. radiator, heating coils in FCU / duct)
4. Chiller
5. Cooling coils in AHU
6. Cooling in space (e.g. chilled beams, cooling coils in FCU)
7. Heat rejection from chiller (e.g. cooling tower, dry air cooling)
8. Heat recovery and / or return air mixing chamber
9. Building Management System (BMS) – controls boilers, chillers, fans, pumps, valves and dampers based on control settings and feedback from sensors

Fig 6.10 Typical components of a conventional HVAC system

Figure 6.11 summarises some of the methods of distributing heating and cooling energy to occupied spaces.[27] These can be configured in various combinations.

It is not unusual to find a mix of different systems in an office building – for example, radiators for perimeter heating, a central AHU providing heating and cooling, and split A/C units retrofitted in meeting rooms for additional localised cooling when required. A mix of systems can provide an energy efficient solution, provided that they are adequately controlled, turned off when not required and avoid fighting each other (i.e. heating and cooling systems do not operate in the same space at the same time).

Radiant and convection

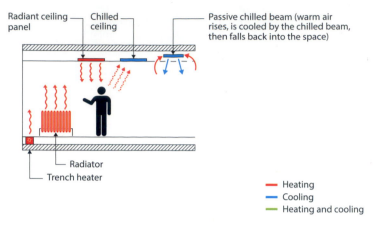

Ducted air supply

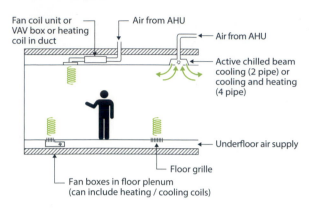

In slab heating/cooling

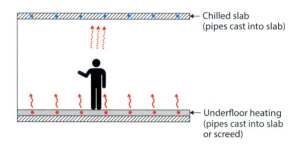

Fan convectors

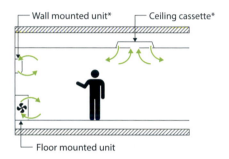

* Typically connected to electric heat pump / VRF system

Fig 6.11 Example methods of delivering heating and cooling to occupants

Variable refrigerant flow (VRF) systems have gained popularity in office buildings since the 1990s, replacing separate water-based heating and cooling systems with a single refrigerant-based system. Appendix H contains a comparison of the key components, advantages and disadvantages of conventional central plant versus VRF.

The systems discussed so far are by no means exhaustive and determining which of the many heating and cooling approaches to use in an office building is beyond the scope of this book.[28]

Reducing heating and cooling energy through design

The following approaches can reduce the heating and cooling energy in new and existing buildings:

- Reduce solar gain in summer and/or heat losses in winter through appropriate façade design.
- Design for typical operation and not just peak loads – systems often run inefficiently at part loads.
- Consider whether thermal mass and night purging could be effective to reduce cooling energy.
- Reduce the volume of fresh (outside) air to be heated or cooled through heat recovery, demand control, ventilation efficiency and pre-occupancy heating/cooling using recycled air.
- Zone systems to suit different thermal and occupancy zones.
- Use energy efficient boilers.
- Design and operate efficient cooling systems considering efficiency of chillers, staging strategy for full and part loads, and raising condenser and chilled water temperatures where possible.
- Use pumps that are efficient at full and part loads and ensure that all pipework is well insulated.

Appendix H provides further guidance on these strategies.

Reducing energy by control

Fundamental to having a low energy heating and cooling system in operation is how it is controlled. The following principles can be considered for most new and existing systems:

- Reduce the set point for heating and increase the set point for cooling – refer to Section 6.2 on thermal comfort and Table 6.5 for a potential seasonal set point strategy.
- Ensure that there is a minimum 4 °C gap between heating and cooling set points to create a comfortable 'dead band' and avoid systems fighting each other, or yo-yoing between heating and cooling.
- Install thermostats away from draughts and heat sources, including direct sunlight.
- In transient spaces, such as meeting rooms, provide a manual on/manual off/absence off control strategy (either a timer or occupancy sensor to turn systems off or down when the space is unoccupied).

- Where radiators are used, install thermostatic radiator valves (TRV) to provide more localised control.
- Provide a zoned out-of-hours heating and cooling control (manual on/manual off/timed off).
- All central heating and cooling plant should be connected to a 7-day timer, with the ability to turn off in holiday periods.
- The controls should be integrated with the ventilation system where this is practical.

Finally, make sure that both the facility manager and the occupants understand how the controls work. Very few people read detailed operations and maintenance manuals (even if they exist) so a simple guide to how the controls work should be provided. Figure 6.12 shows the instructions on the wall next to the VRF system control in Cundall's Manchester office.

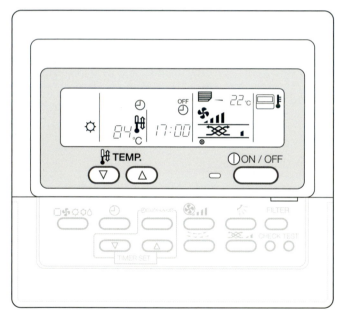

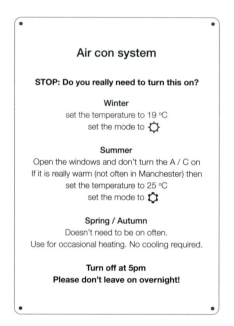

Fig 6.12 Simple guide to using the heating/cooling system – it is rarely turned on because the windows are openable

6.6 LIGHTING

Lighting typically represents around 20% of the operating carbon footprint of an office building. In the Part L/EPC calculations it represents up to 40%,[29] and this weighting clearly encourages more energy efficient lighting and controls. Unfortunately, the calculation is based only on efficiency and not quantity, and so adopting a task-based lighting approach, as described in Section 6.2, is not

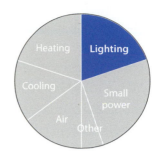

rewarded. In some cases, task lighting (say, 2 W/m²) may be deemed less energy efficient than standard lighting (10 W/m²), even though the energy consumption, by only providing light where it is needed, could be five times lower. This is an example of why simply designing to tick boxes in legislation and rating tools may not lead to the desired low energy outcomes in actual operation.

Lighting design includes providing daylight and electric lighting, and the integration of both, within a space appropriate to the tasks undertaken. Lighting can range from simple lighting systems in a basic fit-out to specialist architectural lighting with bespoke light fittings. The three steps to a low energy lighting design are:

- develop a lighting strategy
- install energy efficient lighting
- set up controls to dim and turn off lights.

The aim should be to achieve a 'lighting energy numeric indicator' (LENI)[30] of not more than 12 kWh/m² per annum. General office lighting installed power should not exceed 10 W/m² with less than 8 W/m² readily achievable for 300 lux lighting in open plan offices.

LIGHTING TERMINOLOGY

The typical terms used in lighting design are:

- **lumens (lm)** – the quantity of light emitted by a lamp
- **lamp efficacy (lm/W)** – the ratio of the lamp output (lumens) and the power it uses (Watts)
- **light output ratio (LOR)** – the ratio of the total light output of a luminaire compared to the total light output of the lamp
- **illuminance (lux)** – is the amount of light reaching a surface measured in lumens per m²
- **colour temperature (kelvin)** – a measure of how warm or cool colours will appear
- **colour rendering index (CRI)** – the extent to which the colours illuminated by a lamp compare to a reference full spectrum lamp on a scale of 1 to 100.

Develop a lighting strategy

It is essential to establish and/or challenge the lighting design brief from the earliest stages, and to obtain building owner/tenant approval if adopting a task lighting approach (refer to Section 6.2). Of critical importance is how daylight and sunlight will be utilised to reduce the hours of operation of artificial lighting and to enhance indoor environment quality. Daylight in design has typically been assessed using daylight factors (the percentage of daylight at a particular location from an overcast sky) but this ignores the dynamic and directional effect of sunlight at different times of the day and year. A better methodology to predict the benefit of daylight, and to test the effectiveness of systems like light shelves, is the Useful Daylight Index.[31]

The integration of daylight, sunlight and artificial lighting will require collaboration with the whole design team as it influences building form, façade design and building services design. As discussed in Section 6.3, sunlight introduces solar heat gains into the building, which can impact on the sizing and energy consumption of mechanical systems and the thermal comfort of occupants. An appropriate balance can usually be found between letting in the sun for daylight and keeping the sun out for thermal comfort.

Issues to consider in developing the lighting strategy include:

- Are spaces with the highest occupancies or lighting requirements located/ orientated to receive maximum daylight and sunlight?
- How will sunlight and daylight be delivered into a space? Consider type, size and orientation of translucent elements (e.g. windows, atria, lightpipes, heliostats, etc.), glare control (e.g. type of blinds) and reflectivity of internal materials (e.g. ceilings, walls).
- Atriums provide visual relief but do not necessarily provide useful daylight to spaces surrounding the atrium – use modelling to confirm whether the atrium will be effective.
- Use contrast to provide visual interest in the space.

Energy efficient lighting

The energy efficiency of a light fitting is a combination of lamp efficacy (lm/W), the luminaire LOR and the power consumption of any ancillary equipment or control gear, such as ballasts or transformers.

Most office buildings currently use fluorescent lighting extensively, with spot lights used as feature lighting, often in meeting rooms and receptions. Spot lights are not an efficient way of providing general lighting, particularly if they use incandescent (halogen) lamps.

Over the past 10 years LEDs have been increasing in efficiency and the cost per lumen has been falling. LEDs have been used primarily for spot lighting, and it was not until 2012 that commercially available LED lighting finally matched the energy efficiency of T5 fluorescent lamps for general office lighting. It may only take a couple of years before the price of these lights is less than T5s, with new entrants to the market cutting costs.

Luminaires have a major influence on the energy efficiency of a lighting system and there are many different designs, including combinations of:

- fixing: recessed, surface mounted or suspended
- glare control: open, louvred or prismatic diffusers
- direction: direct (down) and indirect (upward).

There is little to be gained by putting an efficient lamp in a poor fitting which doesn't distribute the light effectively. It is possible to achieve a 30% reduction in the quantity of luminaires and power density (W/m²) using efficient luminaires effectively. However, the LOR should not be used as the sole selection criteria as the fitting may be directing light to places where it is not useful. Ideally, the measure of lighting efficiency should be based on the efficiency of illuminating the task not the ceiling and floor.

Figure 6.13 illustrates this principle by showing that a super-efficient luminaire may not be the most efficient lighting solution if a large proportion of the light is directed upwards and absorbed by the ceiling. This results in more fittings, capital cost and energy consumption compared to an apparently less efficient luminaire.

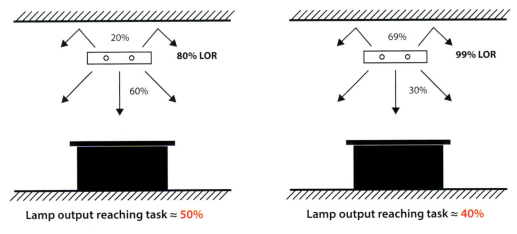

Fig 6.13 An efficient luminaire doesn't necessarily mean efficient lighting

In new office areas an efficient lighting system should be no more than 8 W/m². It is not uncommon to find systems with greater than 25 W/m² in existing buildings. If a new lighting system is not in the refurbishment or fit-out budget then potential improvements may include:

- replacing existing luminaires with new fittings connected to existing wiring
- removing some of the lamps from the fittings (if on separate ballasts) – there is often too much light provided
- replacing old lamps with T5 lamps using conversion kits
- replacing old ballasts with efficient electronic versions
- installing presence detection and daylight dimming to switch off unneeded lights.

For about 20 years it seemed that interior designers couldn't do without halogen downlights and they spread them liberally throughout office buildings like stardust. A 20 m² meeting room with ten 50 W halogen lamps has a power density of 25 W/m². With the improvement in LED technology it should now be possible to avoid using halogen downlights anywhere. In existing buildings opportunities to improve spot lighting efficiency include:

- disconnecting the lights completely (are they actually necessary?)
- removing and replacing with LED spotlights (installing LED lamps into halogen fittings is possible but not as effective or long lasting as purpose-made LED fittings)
- replacing 50 W lamps with 20 W lamps.

Use LED lighting for emergency lights (particularly lights left on 24/7). This will also reduce the battery sizes required.

Lighting controls

The light with the lowest energy consumption is the one that is switched off! Lights are often left on when they are not needed – when there is sufficient daylight or when there is no one in the office. Some simple considerations for control of lighting are:

- Zone lights so that the perimeter can be dimmed or switched off (either manually or by sensors) when there is sufficient daylight.
- Make sure that every light can be manually turned on and off by the building occupants, and add absence off control (linked to a timer or presence detector) where appropriate.

- Avoid lights turning on automatically (unless specifically required for security purposes).
- Label all gang switches so that people know which switch controls each area.
- Position light switches in easily accessible and intuitive locations (e.g. next to doors in cellular rooms).
- Zone lighting circuits to suit occupancy patterns so areas not in use can be easily turned off (either manually or by sensors).

Some modern office buildings have complex computerised lighting control systems with individually addressable lights (refer Figure 6.14). Sometimes these are not necessary and adequate control can be delivered using light switches, timers, presence detectors, daylight dimming and user education. If you do have a complex lighting system then consider the following:

- Is the lighting control system open source or proprietary? If the latter, how easy is it to change settings and modify the system over time? Avoid systems that require a charge-out call if you need to make changes.
- Check how much stand-by power the lighting control system is using when the lights are off. The system may not deliver all the energy savings you thought due to this parasitic load.
- If using desk- or floor-mounted task lights consider connecting these to the overall lighting control system so that they can be automatically turned off out of hours.

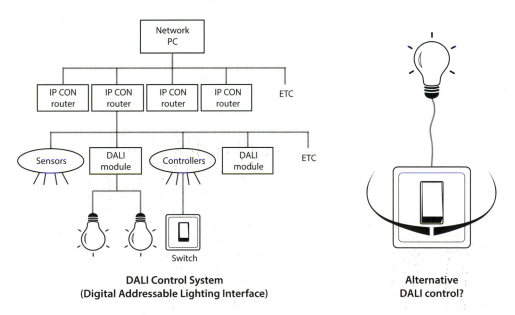

DALI Control System
(Digital Addressable Lighting Interface)

Alternative
DALI control?

Fig 6.14 **DALI lighting controls**

- Provide a simple user guide for control of the lighting system – it might work well in theory but in reality too many lights are left on overnight because a setting was changed or overridden and not subsequently corrected.
- If in doubt – keep it simple.

6.7 PLUG-IN EQUIPMENT

Equipment plugged in by tenants typically accounts for 25% of the operating carbon footprint of offices. It is often referred to as 'small power', and is excluded from Energy Performance Certificates (design rating) but is included in the Display Energy Certificate.

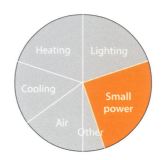

The biggest energy consumer is usually the IT server, which can represent up to 40% of the tenant's electricity consumption. Next are computers, followed by printers/photocopiers and fridges.

Assumptions are made for small power when calculating the electrical capacity and cooling loads in office buildings. This is typically 25 W/m² of NLA, although it is reduced to 15 W/m² in buildings over 1,000 m² to reflect diversity of occupancy and equipment use.[32] In a building with a design occupancy of one person per 10 m² this equates to 150 to 250 W per workstation.

There are three steps to reducing the energy consumption due to plug-in equipment:

1. Only use as much equipment as you need.
2. Select energy efficient equipment.
3. Turn it off when it's not needed.

Turning equipment off

Turning stuff off is not as simple as it sounds. People very rarely switch equipment off at the plug anymore – particularly if it is hidden away in a tangle of cables under the desk. Most IT and domestic equipment, in either stand-by or off modes, draws power. Stand-by power in 2007 was estimated to account for 1% of global CO_2 emissions (for comparison, total air travel accounts for approximately 3%). The One-Watt

Initiative, instigated by the International Energy Agency, aimed to reduce stand-by power use by any appliance to not more than 1 W in 2010, and 0.5 W in 2013.[33] This led to regulation in many countries including the EU, USA and Australia, although it does not cover all of the equipment found in offices, such as photocopiers, servers and plotters. It will also take a few years before old IT equipment, with high stand-by loads, is replaced in all office buildings.

A simple 'time of energy use' study described in Appendix D showed that electricity consumption outside standard working hours accounted for around 50% of the total tenant energy consumption (light and power) in Cundall's offices in 2009. This is because the lights may be left on if a few people work late (or the cleaners are in) and there is some equipment that cannot be turned off at night and weekends, such as servers and fridges.

Figure 6.15 shows how the breakdown of small power energy consumption in a typical office might look.[34] Figure 6.16 (overleaf) shows the breakdown of energy consumption by item. The two charts illustrate which battles to pick to make noticeable reductions. While unplugging phone chargers is easy, they have negligible energy consumption – it is the server room, computers and monitors which offer the largest savings, accounting for around 90% of an occupant's small power energy.

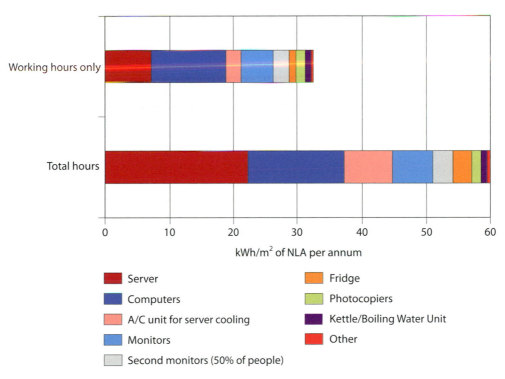

Fig 6.15 Typical office equipment energy consumption (with efficient stand-by mode enabled)

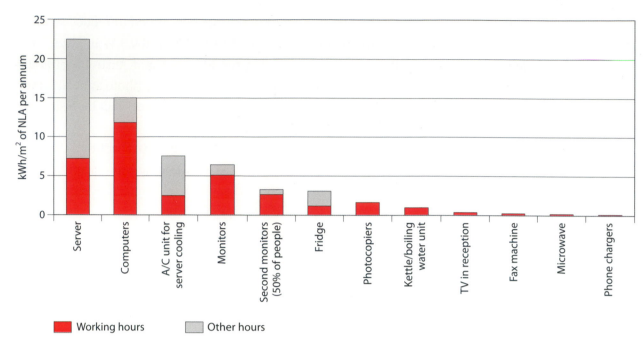

Fig 6.16 Breakdown of typical office equipment energy consumption (with efficient stand-by mode enabled)

Servers

Servers present the biggest and most difficult issue to tackle, mainly because you can't turn the server off at night – it runs 8,760 hours a year. The IT industry has started to take steps towards improving the efficiency of servers, and all the other equipment that goes into the server rack, including switches, UPS, back-up systems and so on.

Newer virtual servers reduce energy consumption when demand for processing reduces (e.g. at night or weekends). This is like taking your foot off the accelerator pedal in a car when you want to go slower; with old servers the energy consumption was constant, even when little processing was required (like keeping the engine at full revs while waiting at the traffic lights).

Many IT functions are now outsourced to servers in remote data centres. While this reduces energy consumption in the office building, it is only transferring the associated CO_2e emissions to another location. The theory is that the data centres, by concentrating activity in purpose-built facilities, will be able to provide the IT function in a more energy efficient manner, particularly the cooling component. This depends on the data centre used, as performance can vary significantly and unfortunately many are not very energy efficient.[35]

Computers and monitors

If the power management features of computers and monitors are not enabled this can lead to excessive energy consumption, particularly if people don't turn off their computers and monitors at night. Figure 6.17 shows the difference that a good power management strategy can make (based on a 100 W PC/monitor, a stand-by load of 7 W, and an occupancy of one per 10 m^2). The poor strategy assumes the PC and monitors do not switch to stand-by except on weekends.

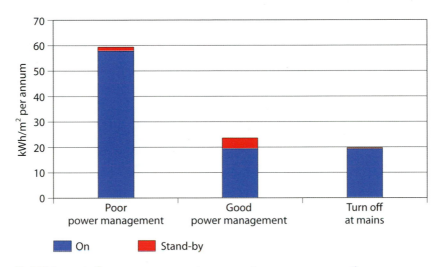

Fig 6.17 **Impact of power management on computer energy consumption**

Implementing good power management policies alone, with no compromise on productivity, could save 60% of the electricity consumed at each workstation. Switching off at the mains would save a further 10%.

Energy saving initiatives to consider include:

- purchasing computers and monitors which:
  - consume a maximum of 1 W in stand-by/off modes
  - exceed the latest Energy Star requirements
  - have a high processing performance to energy consumption ratio (a PC can be energy efficient but slow)
- getting the IT department to implement power management strategies:
  - switching equipment off at night (rather than leaving it on overnight for software upgrades)
  - establishing sleep and hibernation power management settings as a corporate standard

- making it easy to switch off equipment at the plug – providing an accessible on/off switch so that all power can be turned off without crawling under the desk.

Similar strategies apply to printers, plotters and photocopiers connected to the IT system.

THIN CLIENTS

Like the old mainframe computer systems, thin client or blade PCs, use a central server for all the processing with only a small terminal box and monitor at the workstation. The benefit is that the heat generated by the servers is concentrated in one space (and so can be dealt with more efficiently) and the internal heat gain in the main office space is reduced. This may then enable more energy efficient cooling options of the office space to become viable, including natural ventilation.

Other equipment

Some other ways to reduce small power energy consumption include:

- selecting the most energy efficient appliances available based on energy rating labels
- taking into account the fact that fridges are more efficient if they have adequate ventilation clearance to back and sides
- installing boiling water units with timers to turn off outside normal hours; if you need a cup of tea at 2 a.m. on Sunday morning then use a kettle
- switching printers off at night
- reducing the number of printers in the office
- discouraging the use of electric convector heaters under desks – try to solve any local thermal discomfort issues by tackling the root cause (e.g. draughts, poor controls/zoning, inappropriate winter clothing).

6.8 OTHER BUILDING SERVICES

The following systems account for around 5% of the operating carbon footprint of typical office buildings:

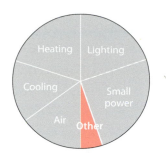

- domestic hot water
- lifts
- external lighting.

The lighting and ventilation due to underground car parking can add a further 2 to 5% to the total carbon footprint. Commercial kitchens and staff cafes, which can sometimes be included in large corporate office buildings, can add another 5 to 10%. The electrical power supply to the building also has an influence on carbon emissions.

Domestic hot water

Office buildings use relatively little domestic hot water (DHW), the main uses being wash hand basins, tea rooms and showers. A typical UK benchmark for DHW use in offices is 6 kWh/m^2 (central gas) or 4 kWh/m^2 (local electric). In Australia, the NABERS Energy Guide to Building Energy Estimation suggests 2 kWh/m^2 of NLA. If the building has specialist catering facilities then demand will be higher.

To reduce the CO_2e emissions associated with DHW, consider:

- reducing water consumption by:
    - determining whether hot water taps are required to wash hand basins
    - installing water efficient taps (<4 l/min) and showers (<9 l/min)
    - retrofitting in-line flow restrictors (these work better than aerators and don't damage the tap fitting) or turning down the isolator valve to reduce flow
    - fixing any water leaks
- reviewing whether point-of-use hot water generation (electric showers and hot water sink units) will be more energy efficient than generating hot water centrally and then pumping around the building[36]
- if using a central DHW system then:
    - insulating all domestic hot water pipework
    - minimising dead legs
    - considering solar thermal or waste heat from chillers to preheat water
- utilising heat recovery systems for showers – these extract heat from the shower waste water pipe to preheat the cold water supply to the shower and/ or DHW storage tank (calorifier).

Lifts

Lifts are excluded from EPC ratings in the UK. The NABERS Energy Simulation Protocol sets 8 kWh/m^2 of NLA as representing typical lift energy use in Australian office buildings. This is equivalent to 4 kgCO$_2$e/m^2 of GIA in the UK.

Strategies to reduce lift energy consumption include:

- using the stairs – make these easy to access, highly visible and attractive to use, particularly in buildings less than ten storeys high
- minimising the number of lifts required (use modelling and advanced controls to justify – this saves capital, energy and maintenance costs)
- installing efficient variable voltage variable frequency (VVVF) electric motors instead of hydraulics
- using regenerative drives which store energy when braking
- programming lifts to minimise lift movements and avoid ghosting (moving up and down the building when no one is using them)
- turning off individual or groups of lifts during non-peak periods
- installing efficient lights in lifts with PIR control.

External lighting

Generally, the same principles discussed in Section 6.6 apply to external lighting. The key issues to consider are:

- selecting efficient lamps and luminaires with a minimum output of 80 lumens/watt
- lighting the task or feature only and avoiding lights with an uplighting component
- providing timers, motion detectors and/or daylight sensors.

LED lamps are a good choice for external street lighting, particularly when the LED is bonded directly to the outer casing. LEDs need a good heat sink, and the exposed metal casing in the middle of winter, when the lights are on the most, is effective at dissipating heat.

A key issue with external lighting is to avoid night sky pollution. Apart from the environmental impacts, illuminating the sky is clearly a waste of light and therefore energy.

Car park lighting and ventilation

The energy consumption of mechanically ventilated underground car parking is excluded from EPC ratings. To reduce energy consumption associated with car parks in office buildings:

- design lighting systems to a maximum 2 W/m²
- install presence detectors to turn most lights off – leaving a minimum lighting level for security
- paint ceilings and walls white (or use light-coloured concrete) to improve uniformity of lighting
- use natural ventilation whenever possible
- control mechanical ventilation systems with carbon monoxide (CO) sensors
- use impulse fans instead of ducted systems on large floor plates.

ENERGY SAVINGS IN THE BUILDING POWER SUPPLY

The power supply to the building influences the electricity consumption of the whole building. Most large buildings and multi-building sites are connected to a high voltage power supply and require a transformer to reduce the voltage. These typically incur 1% losses, which increase at low loadings. Selecting the most efficient transformer possible and avoiding oversizing will reduce CO_2e emissions.

The total power (kVA) is the product of voltage (volts) and current (amps). However, the actual power (kW) is less than this due to the effect of inductive loads, caused by the generation of magnetic fields in equipment such as motors, compressors in heat pumps and chillers, and fluorescent lighting. The power factor is a measure of how efficiently electrical power is consumed:

actual power (kW) = total power (kVA) × power factor

A power factor of less than one means that some power is being 'lost' due to the inductive effects – the current is lagging the voltage. Power factor correction is achieved by adding capacitors to the electrical circuit to make the current lead the voltage, balancing out the inductive effect. An average power factor of 0.95 (i.e. 5% losses) in a building is usually considered to be good practice.

Voltage optimisation has been wideley promoted as a simple energy saving device which connects to a building's power supply to reduce the voltage. The standard

continued overleaf

continued

voltage for the European Union is 230 V which, with tolerances, can vary between 215 and 250 V. Voltage typically varies across the UK between 220 and 240 V. Most equipment in the EU should be designed to operate at 230 V but some older equipment in the UK was designed for 240 V while in Europe it was 220 V.

As discussed above, power = voltage × current. However, reducing the voltage does not necessarily reduce the energy consumption of all equipment. For example, if the voltage is reduced it just takes longer for a kettle to boil. Energy savings can be achieved in older lighting systems because reducing the voltage makes the lights become dimmer, thereby reducing consumption.

The energy reduction benefit of voltage optimisation devices is highly dependent on the type of electrical equipment in a building. Modern buildings will see little benefit. However, office buildings with old lighting and motors could achieve electrical savings of between 5 and 10%. A detailed site survey is essential to determine if there will be any measurable benefit using these systems.

6.9 COMMISSIONING, HANDOVER AND MAINTENANCE

If you purchase a new car you would expect all the systems to be working and a simple user manual to be included at handover. You would also expect to have to take the car in for regular servicing and perform routine maintenance (such as keeping the tyres inflated), in order for the car to run efficiently, and to keep working reliably as it gets older. The same should apply to buildings. Unfortunately, many buildings are poorly commissioned, have minimal guides for users and are irregularly serviced.

On paper, most new buildings are energy efficient. As discussed in Chapter 2 and Section 6.1, the reality is less encouraging.

Commissioning

The importance of correct commissioning is recognised in all the major rating tools, such as LEED, BREEAM and Green Star, and reference is usually made to CIBSE, BSRIA or ASHRAE commissioning guides. On many projects commissioning is left to the last minute, as illustrated in Figure 6.18, because it is considered compressible or is not properly planned or both.

The commissioning process should ideally start in the early design stages and continue beyond handover to include seasonal commissioning and fine tuning of

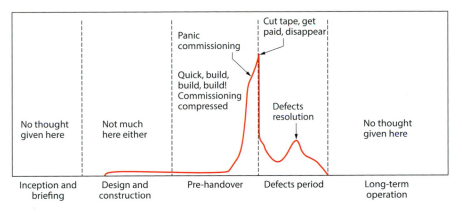

Fig 6.18 How commissioning is often carried out on projects (source: Roderic Bunn, BSRIA)

systems. This is because, despite good intentions, systems rarely work properly on day one and buildings can't fix themselves. As buildings and control systems become more complex, implementing a detailed commissioning process becomes even more important. Buildings with fully integrated ICT and controls networks require considerable attention to detail and coordination between suppliers, installers and commissioning/controls contractors to ensure that all the systems work correctly and integrate with each other, not just at handover but also in the future when individual systems are modified. Appendix H provides some guidance on this.

Handover and post occupancy evaluation (POE)

Designers and constructors of buildings rarely do the following:

1 Handover the building to the client with clear instructions and training on how it is supposed to work.
2 Stay involved during the initial occupancy period to fine-tune any teething problems.
3 Go back into the building at a later date to find out how it is actually working and then:
    – assist in fixing any problems
    – apply any lessons learnt (what worked, what didn't) to future building design.

Items 2 and 3 are often not due to a lack of interest, but because there is usually no contractual obligation to do so, and consequently no fees allocated to perform these tasks after handover.

The Soft Landings Framework[37] was established in the UK to provide a structure for project teams to stay engaged, hand-holding the client during the first months of operation to fine-tune and de-bug systems and ensure that the occupiers understand how to control and make best use of their new work environment. Table 6.6 shows the five key stages of the framework.

	Stage	Description
1	Inception and briefing	Allow more time for constructive dialogue between the designer, constructor and client
2	Design development and review	Bring the entire project team together to review insights from comparable projects and detail how the building will work from the point of view of the manager and individual user
3	Pre-handover	Enable operators to spend more time on understanding interfaces and systems before occupation
4	Initial aftercare	Continuing involvement by the client, design and building team benefiting from lessons learned and occupant satisfaction surveys
5	Years 1–3 extended aftercare and post-occupancy evaluation	Complete the virtuous circle for future projects, to close the loop between design expectation and reality

Table 6.6 The five key stages of the Soft Landings Framework (source: BSRIA, 2009)

With increasing awareness of the performance gap between design and reality, the use of the Soft Landings Framework and post-occupancy evaluation[38] will hopefully start to gain momentum. Making these mandatory in the contracts for designers and contractors would be a good start. The UK government has indicated it intends to do so for public buildings from 2016 onwards.

Maintenance

Building maintenance is not glamorous and is often focused on avoiding failure rather than improving efficiency. Inadequate maintenance can have a detrimental impact on the energy performance of buildings.

The key elements to the maintenance of building fabric and building services are:

- design the systems so that they are accessible for safe maintenance[39]
- establish and implement a maintenance plan
- comply with relevant legislation, including mandatory air conditioning and F-gas inspections in the EU.[40]

6.10 PEOPLE

A common mistake that people make when trying to design something completely foolproof is to underestimate the ingenuity of complete fools.
Douglas Adams

People in buildings are a nuisance. They complain about the conditions – too hot, too cold, too draughty, too stuffy – then mess up the controls when they try to fix the problem. If buildings didn't have occupants they would work perfectly.[41]

To make a building work successfully requires the cooperation or buy-in of the occupants and the facility managers, which at some point involves communicating the operational strategies. The key requirements are:

- keep it simple
- make it easy to do the right thing
- label controls clearly
- provide user guides where appropriate.

Controls

Things should be made as simple as possible, but not simpler.
Albert Einstein

Controls are critical to energy performance, but do not have to be complex to be effective. This was discussed in previous sections in this chapter.

In developing a controls strategy for a new or refurbished building the designers should first agree with the client who will control the building and how this will be managed. Once a strategy has been agreed it is important that a clear description of how the system is intended to work is passed on to both the contractor and the occupants.

In owner-occupied buildings, or where the tenant is known, engaging with the building occupants early in the design process should be encouraged and not feared. The typical process of having one person, usually a senior manager, representing all users will often result in a conservative solution, particularly if they haven't really discussed the opportunities with the rest of the occupants' business.

User guides

User guides should be tailored to suit the audience: facility managers need more detail than a typical occupant who just wants to know which button to press or who to contact to change a setting. An analogy is the 'Getting Started' one page guide that comes with a new laptop or TV, which is usually the only document anyone reads. The detailed manual rarely gets opened unless you want to do something unusual, or the thing has stopped working.

Tenant fit-out guides

Many office buildings are built to either shell and core or Category A fit-out (ceiling, lighting, HVAC and carpet) standards by the developer. The tenant then undertakes their own fit-out. From an environmental perspective it is usually preferable in speculative offices to build to shell and core to avoid tenants ripping out the new lighting and carpets installed by the landlord and sending these to landfill.

In either case, the landlord should provide fit-out guidelines for the tenant explaining how the building works, detailing fit-out requirements to avoid a reduction in the performance of the building systems, and specifying measures that the tenants can or should take to reduce energy consumption. Examples include:

- partition layouts to suit zoning of HVAC systems and to avoid blocking air-flow paths in naturally ventilated or mixed mode buildings
- zoning of lighting and the potential to adopt a task lighting approach
- exhaust of photocopier rooms/zones
- cooling of server rooms
- connection of tenant cooling systems to base building chilled or condenser water circuits.

Green teams

Landlords can encourage tenants to establish green teams to look at ways in which the occupants can reduce the environmental impact of their operations. In multi-tenanted buildings the landlord could facilitate quarterly meetings of the green team leaders to encourage knowledge sharing between different organisations in the same building.

A good framework to guide green team activities is the One Planet Living initiative (refer to Table 6.7) developed by BioRegional and the World Wide Fund for Nature.[42]

Principle	Objective
Zero carbon	Making buildings more energy efficient and delivering all energy with renewable technologies
Zero waste	Reducing waste, reusing where possible, and ultimately sending zero waste to landfill
Sustainable transport	Encouraging low carbon modes of transport to reduce emissions, and reducing the need to travel
Sustainable materials	Using and selling sustainable products that have low embodied energy
Local and sustainable food	Choosing low impact, local, seasonal and organic diets and reducing food waste
Sustainable water	Reducing water usage in buildings and in the products we buy; preventing flooding and pollution
Land use and wildlife	Protecting and expanding existing natural habitats and creating new spaces for wildlife
Culture and heritage	Reviving local identity and wisdom; supporting and participating in the arts
Equity and local economy	Creating local economies that support fair employment and international fair trade
Health and happiness	Encouraging active, sociable, meaningful lives to promote good health and well-being

Table 6.7 The ten One Planet Living principles (source: BioRegional/WWF)

6.11 SUMMARY

> *Unmanageable complication is the enemy of good performance. So why are we making buildings technically and bureaucratically complicated in the name of sustainability, when we can't get the simple things right?*
> Bill Bordass OBE, Usable Buildings Trust

This chapter has set out a framework of ten steps to systematically tackle energy consumption in new and existing buildings. These are summarised in Table 6.8 (overleaf). Further details are provided in Appendix H.

Every building is unique – a combination of location, layout, façade, systems and occupants – and consequently there is no one-size-fits-all approach to reducing energy consumption. Different buildings will require different solutions within the ten steps.

One of the biggest barriers to change and innovation within the property industry is the number of parties involved, the complexity of procurement contracts and getting everyone aligned to achieve common goals (refer to Figure 6.19 on page 131). Procurement contracts for designers and contractors rarely provide any incentive for

Issue	Key points
1 Understand how energy is being used	Compare the performance against benchmarks, focus on operational energy not design ratings, identify the big energy uses and users and target these. Establish a metering and energy management plan. If you can't monitor it, you can't manage it.
2 Challenge design criteria	Consider whether alternative lighting and thermal comfort criteria can be adopted – task lighting approach and wider temperature bands.
3 Building fabric	Achieve an appropriate balance between daylight, views, heat loss and solar gain – is a fully glazed building the best solution? Provide good air tightness.
4 Ventilation	Can the windows be opened and a natural/mixed mode strategy be adopted? Mechanical systems should be designed to minimise fan power and running hours.
5 Heating and cooling	Design systems for efficient year-round operation and not just to meet peak demand. Zoning and controls are critical.
6 Lighting	Provide the right amount of light only where and when it's needed. Develop a lighting strategy using daylight, efficient fittings and controls.
7 Equipment	Purchase energy efficient servers, computers, monitors and appliances. Implement power management strategies and turn stuff off at night.
8 Other services	Saving water saves energy. Use efficient lifts and reduce unnecessary lift movement. Consider power factor correction.
9 Commissioning, handover and maintenance	Implement a commissioning plan and use the Soft Landings Framework. Incentivise the project team beyond handover. Proactive maintenance saves energy.
10 People	Engage with occupants and make it easy for them to save energy. Establish green teams and provide simple user guides.

Table 6.8 Summary of the ten steps to reducing energy consumption

operational efficiency, and the tenant lease agreements usually contain little mention of cooperation between parties to achieve energy savings.

Owner occupied buildings tend to be more innovative because investment in energy efficiency by the owner results in cost savings for the owner. In commercial buildings, unless the tenant will pay extra rent, it is often difficult for landlords or developers to justify the investment in energy reduction. This issue is discussed further in Chapter 10 – Making the business case.

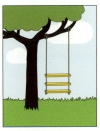 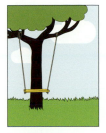 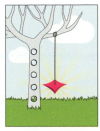 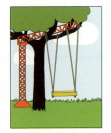 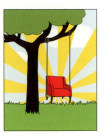

How the customer explained it | How the project manager briefed it | How the architect designed it | How the engineer designed it | How the agent marketed it

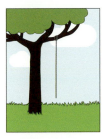 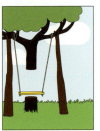 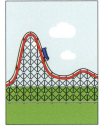 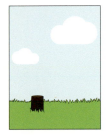 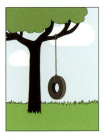

What was proposed after value engineering | What the contractor finally built | How the customer was billed | How it was supported after handover | What the customer really needed

Fig 6.19 **The delivery process for buildings?**

**Keep it simple, size it right,
do it well, follow it through,
tune it up, capture the feedback and
continuously improve.**

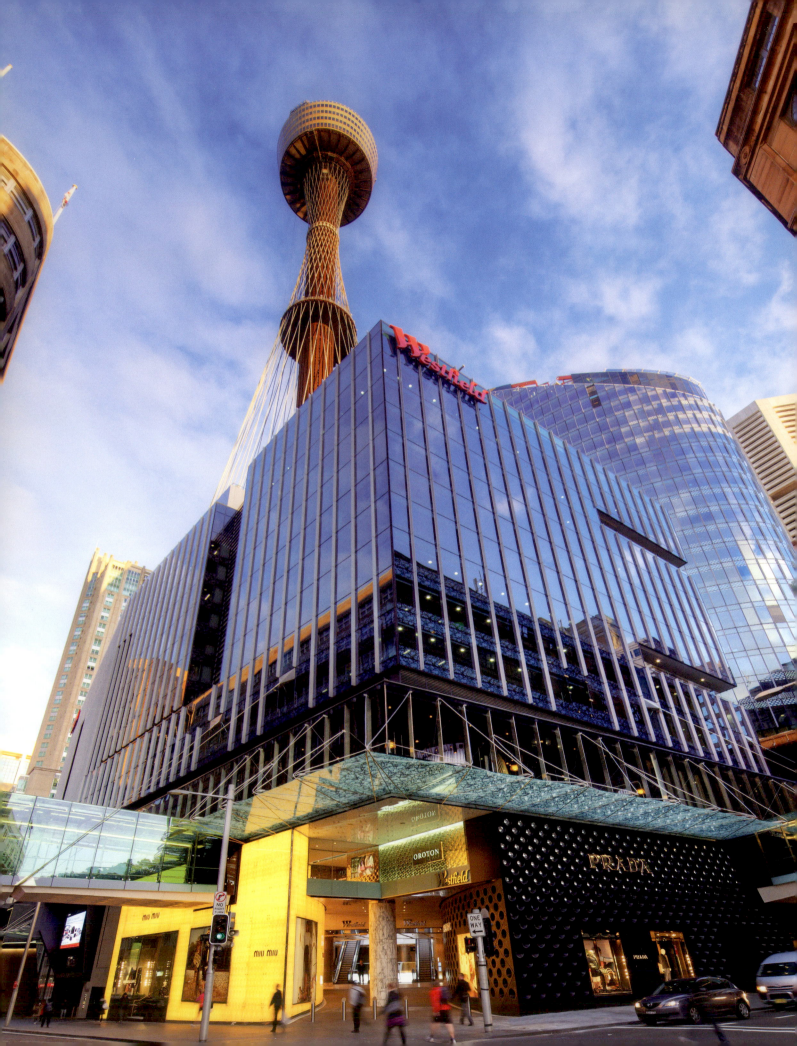

Chapter 7

Renewable energy

I've come up with a set of rules that describe our reactions to technologies:
1. *Anything that is in the world when you're born is normal and ordinary and is just a natural part of the way the world works.*
2. *Anything that's invented between when you're fifteen and thirty-five is new and exciting and revolutionary and you can probably get a career in it.*
3. *Anything invented after you're thirty-five is against the natural order of things.*

Douglas Adams

The Salmon of Doubt, Harmony Books, New York, 2002

This chapter assesses the energy and CO_2e savings that renewable (and low carbon) energy systems can make in individual buildings and highlights the key issues to consider when analysing and selecting appropriate systems.

There are many motivations to install renewable energy systems on, or in, buildings including: obtaining planning approval,[1] scoring points in rating tools, increasing security/diversity of energy supply, publically displaying corporate environmental commitment, and getting a financial investment return, particularly if there are government incentives available. Sometimes the driver is to reduce the carbon footprint.

A number of countries intend to introduce 'nearly zero energy' or 'zero carbon' building legislation by 2020, and on-site renewable energy is seen as a key component in achieving this.[2] As this chapter will show, most urban commercial buildings cannot become zero carbon using on-site systems and investment in large scale off-site renewables will be required to make up the difference.

7.1 TYPES OF RENEWABLE ENERGY SYSTEMS

Renewable systems can generate the two forms of energy used in buildings:

- **heat** – a low grade energy that is usually generated at the point of use, either in buildings or in district heating networks
- **electricity** – a high grade energy that can be generated anywhere and distributed via national grid infrastructure.

Since heat is difficult to move around (district heating systems are rare in many countries) and demand for heat is seasonal (higher in winter, lower in summer) then any surplus heat generated by renewable heat systems in individual buildings is usually wasted. The heating systems evaluated in this chapter are:

- solar thermal
- heat pumps
- biomass boilers
- combined heat and power (CHP).

In comparison, any surplus electricity generated on site can usually be exported into the national grid and so doesn't go to waste. Renewable electricity systems can therefore be sized to suit available space and budget whereas renewable heating systems are usually sized to suit the building's heat demand. The electrical systems evaluated are:

- photovoltaics
- wind turbines
- combined heat and power (CHP).

The evaluation of CHP is for both natural gas and biofuel, and includes trigeneration (the provision of cooling as well as heating). There are many other renewable energy systems available which are not covered in this book as they are rarely used in commercial office buildings in the UK. These include solar air heating, cooling from solar thermal, geothermal heating, tidal power and hydro-electric.

RENEWABLE VERSUS LOW CARBON

Renewable and low carbon energy systems are terms that are often used interchangeably but actually mean two different things:

- **Renewable systems** use a source of energy that can be replenished at the same rate that it is used. This includes wind, sun and biomass (assuming that demand for biomass fuel does not outstrip supply).
- **Low carbon systems** produce energy (heat or electricity) with much lower greenhouse gas emissions than conventional fossil fuel systems.

A system can be low carbon but not renewable, such as a natural gas CHP. Conversely, a biofuel CHP can be renewable but not necessarily low carbon – it depends on the biofuel used. This is discussed later in the chapter.

7.2 CALCULATING THE ENERGY, CO_2e AND COST SAVINGS

Every building is unique in its location, size, energy profile and available space for renewables. The contribution that renewables can make in any building will therefore vary. The methodologies described in this book can be used during feasibility studies to estimate the potential energy and carbon savings in new and existing buildings.

The heating energy demand in buildings varies quite significantly depending on the building type, occupant intensity and activity, façade performance, operating hours, fresh air quantities and whether heat recovery systems are installed. New office buildings, with efficient façades, heat recovery systems and intensive internal activity (lights, people and equipment) can require little space heating and have limited demand for domestic hot water (DHW). Older buildings with leaky façades tend to have higher heating consumption. In warmer countries than the UK the demand for heating can be relatively minor.

While this book focuses on office buildings, due to their relatively low demand for annual heating and DHW the contribution of renewable heating systems can be small. To allow the viability of these systems to be considered in a broader context, their use in a hotel is also evaluated. Hotels have a much higher heat energy consumption, due to space heating (the building is occupied 24/7) and high levels of domestic hot water use (showers and kitchens). If the hotel has a swimming pool then heat energy consumption is higher still.

Buildings X and Hotel Y

Table 7.1 (overleaf) summarises the annual energy performance of two typical building types in the UK – a commercial office (Building X) and a hotel (Hotel Y) – which will be used to evaluate the CO_2e and cost benefits of different renewable energy systems. The floor area and total CO_2e emissions for the two example buildings are identical – the difference is in the split of electricity to gas energy consumption.

Figure 7.1 shows the seasonal heating energy demand profiles used in the evaluation of the renewable heating systems. Further details on the energy profiles of these hypothetical buildings are given in Appendix M.

To estimate the energy and CO_2e savings due to renewable heating systems, the base case assumes that all heat in the buildings is provided from natural gas boilers with an efficiency of 90%. This means that 100 kWh of gas energy is converted into 90 kWh of heat.

The embodied carbon of the systems, and how many years it takes for the energy generated to offset this, is not considered in this chapter.

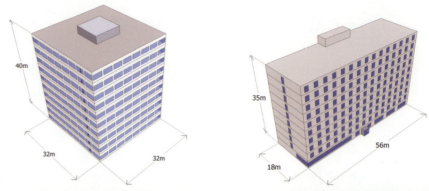

	Building X			Hotel Y		
Gross internal area (m²)	10,000			10,000		
Electricity to gas energy split	67:33			31:69		
	Electricity	Gas	**Total**	Electricity	Gas	**Total**
Energy consumption (kWh/m²)	150	75	**225**	100	225	**325**
Energy costs (£/m²)	£15	£2.6	**£17.6**	£10	£7.9	**£17.9**
CO_2 emissions (kgCO_2e/m²)	90	15	**105**	60	45	**105**
Primary energy (kWh/m²)	405	83	**488**	270	248	**518**
Indicative DEC rating	F			D		

Table 7.1 Summary of Building X and Hotel Y base case annual energy, CO_2e and costs

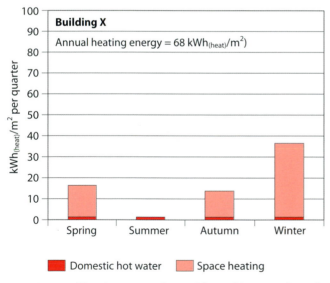
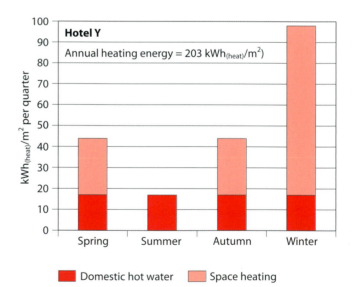

Fig 7.1 Seasonal heating energy demand for Building X and Hotel Y

Percentage of operating energy

The contribution of renewable energy is often obscured by expressing the benefits as a percentage of the building's design energy consumption. The percentage is typically based on comparing predicted renewable energy outputs (which are often higher than reality) with modelled energy consumption (which is usually substantially lower). This results in a stated contribution which sounds impressive but is often misleading. The property industry needs to agree a common method of expressing the contribution of renewable energy in real terms. In this chapter the contributions are expressed in $kgCO_2e/m^2$ of GIA and percentage reductions in operating (not design) carbon.

Costs

Any evaluation of renewable energy systems needs to consider both capital and operating costs – and any book that tries to do so will always get it wrong because these costs can fluctuate rapidly, particularly when government incentives are introduced (or removed). The costs used in this chapter are indicative of prices for large commercial buildings in the UK at the start of 2013. Table 7.2 shows the tariffs assumed for different energy sources, together with the CO_2e emission factors.[3] Energy costs change each year, with prices generally rising while grid electricity CO_2e emissions gradually decrease.

	Energy tariff (including VAT)	Calorific value	Energy cost p/kWh	$kgCO_2e/kWh$
Grid electricity	–	–	10	0.60
Natural gas	–	–	3.5	0.20
Heating oil	60p/litre	9.8 kWh/litre	6.0	0.31
LPG	50p/litre	6.6 kWh/litre	7.6	0.26
Wood pellet	£220/tonne	4.8 kWh/kg	4.6	0.04
Wood chip (30% MC)*	£100/tonne	3.5 kWh/kg	2.9	0.02
Biofuel	–	–	7.0	0.12**

* MC = moisture content. Refer to Appendix I for details.

** This can vary from 0.06 $kgCO_2e/kWh$ (recycled cooking oil) to over 0.5 $kgCO_2e/kWh$ – refer to Appendix B for details.

Table 7.2 Typical costs and CO_2e factors for energy sources in the UK

It is assumed that the buildings are connected to the national grid and that any surplus electricity generated can be exported to the grid. Exporting electricity does not affect the CO_2e saving (the electricity is not being wasted) but does impact on the financial evaluation. This is because electricity tariffs vary by time of use (weekends and evenings are usually cheaper) and export tariffs are lower than consumption tariffs (electricity companies do not buy electricity from you at the same rate that they sell it back). In this book a flat rate of 10p/kWh is adopted and all electricity is assumed to be used in the building (i.e. not exported). This gives a best case scenario for the production of electricity – the actual energy cost savings will be lower when off-peak tariffs and exporting surplus electricity to the grid are taken into account.

The analysis of operating costs in this chapter excludes any additional maintenance costs which would also need to be added to the financial evaluation. The benefit of any government incentives for renewables, such as feed-in tariffs for photovoltaic panels, are also excluded as the rules and payments for these can, and do, change abruptly.[4]

Financial evaluation of renewable systems

The most common type of financial evaluation is the simple payback period. This is the number of years taken for the energy cost savings to equal the initial capital cost:

$$\text{payback period (years)} = \frac{\text{capital cost}}{\text{annual energy cost saving}}$$

A payback of less than 5 years is usually considered to be reasonable for investment in energy cost savings in most buildings. A payback of up to 10 years might be acceptable to an owner-occupier but in most commercial buildings this is a long time to recover the initial investment, and is also longer than the average tenancy lease in the UK.[5]

The payback period, while very simple, does not reflect the value of money over time or the cost per tonne of CO_2e saved. Is it better to make a large initial investment that will provide energy savings over time, or to put in a lower cost system that will have higher annual energy costs?

To answer this question requires consideration of net present cost (NPC),[6] which uses a discount rate to estimate the value of revenue and costs in the future based on inflation, interest rates, cost of finance and risk. The line from one of Aesop's fables 'a bird in the hand is worth two in the bush' applies equally to money – would you rather have £1 in the bank today or the promise of £1 in the bank in 10 years' time? In this chapter a discount rate of 5% is used (meaning the promised £1, ten years hence, is worth 61p today). The cost of energy will also increase over time and a conservative estimate of 3% per annum above inflation is assumed. The net present cost of a system depends on the timeframe that the investment is considered over. In this chapter 15 years is adopted as the time span.

Finally, the cost of carbon (£ per tCO_2e) for each system is estimated. This is based on the net present cost of the system over 15 years divided by the total CO_2e emissions saved over the same period.

$$\text{cost of carbon (£/}tCO_2e\text{: 15 years @ 5\%)} = \frac{\text{net present cost over 15 years @ 5\% discount rate}}{tCO_2e \text{ saved per year} \times 15 \text{ years}}$$

To put this value into perspective, the cost of carbon is typically between £10 to £20 per tonne of CO_2 under various carbon tax, emission trading schemes and carbon offset programs.

7.3 SOLAR THERMAL

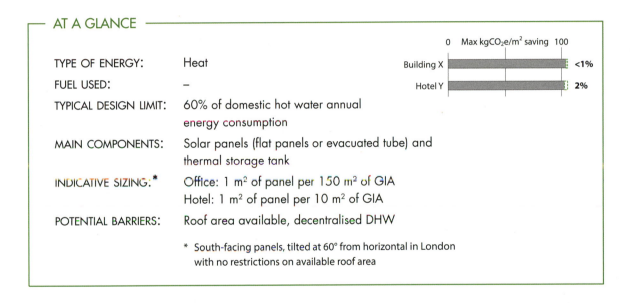

AT A GLANCE

			0 Max $kgCO_2e/m^2$ saving 100
TYPE OF ENERGY:	Heat		Building X <1%
FUEL USED:	–		Hotel Y 2%
TYPICAL DESIGN LIMIT:	60% of domestic hot water annual energy consumption		
MAIN COMPONENTS:	Solar panels (flat panels or evacuated tube) and thermal storage tank		
INDICATIVE SIZING:*	Office: 1 m² of panel per 150 m² of GIA Hotel: 1 m² of panel per 10 m² of GIA		
POTENTIAL BARRIERS:	Roof area available, decentralised DHW		

* South-facing panels, tilted at 60° from horizontal in London with no restrictions on available roof area

Solar thermal collectors convert solar radiation energy into heat energy with an average annual efficiency of between 30 and 50% (refer to Figure 7.2 overleaf). There are two main types available: flat plate and evacuated tube collectors, which both have similar levels of efficiency when considered on a gross panel area.[7] Solar thermal systems are ideal for domestic hot water (DHW) systems as these have a near-constant daily demand for heat all year round. They are less suitable for space heating because the sun doesn't shine enough in winter, when most heat is required.

The systems are typically sized to supply about 60% of the annual DHW demand with the remainder provided by a boiler or other heat source. In the summer they can provide most of the DHW demand but this drops off significantly in the winter. If they were sized for 90% of the annual energy demand then the system would need to be over twice the size and approximately one-third of the heat generated would be rejected and go to waste.[8]

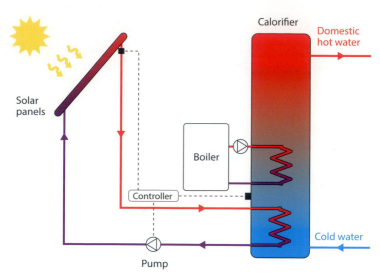

Fig 7.2 Typical components of a DHW solar thermal system

Solar thermal on Building X and Hotel Y

The calculation below illustrates a quick method of determining the size of a typical system and the resulting reduction in the building's CO_2e emissions. To estimate the area of panels, the following needs to be considered:

- the annual solar irradiation on each panel of the building (the amount of solar energy, in kWh/m^2, received by a panel based on its location, orientation and tilt)
- the efficiency of the panels in converting solar energy into useful heat
- system losses in pipework and storage tanks
- the demand for DHW in the building.

A simple calculation for the annual heat output from a typical solar thermal system is:

mean solar irradiation[9] on south facing panel inclined at 60° in London
    = 1,078 kWh/m^2
annual average efficiency based on gross collector area = 40% (assumed)
assumed system losses = 3%
annual heat output per m^2 of panel = 1,078 × 40% × (1 - 0.03)
    = 418 kWh/m^2

The total energy generated by a solar thermal system should provide 60% of the annual DHW energy consumption. Table 7.3 summarises the calculation for Building X and Hotel Y, assuming that the gas boilers have an efficiency of 90% and the natural gas CO_2e emission factor is 0.2 kgCO_2e/kWh.

		Unit	Calculation	Building X	Hotel Y
(A)	Solar system output	$kWh_{(heat)}/m^2$		418	
(B)	Annual DHW demand	$kWh_{(heat)}$		45,000	675,000
(C)	60% of DHW demand by solar	$kWh_{(heat)}$	$= 0.6 \times B$	27,000	405,000
(D)	**Area of panels required**	**m^2**	$= C/A$	**65**	**969**
(E)	Heat from gas boilers (40%)	$kWh_{(heat)}$	$= B - C$	18,000	270,000
(F)	Gas consumption of boiler	kWh	$= E/0.9$	20,000	300,000
(G)	Gas consumption without solar	kWh	$= B/0.9$	50,000	750,000
(H)	Reduction in gas consumption	kWh	$= G - F$	30,000	450,000
(I)	Total reduction in CO_2e	$kgCO_2e$	$= H \times 0.2$	6,000	90,000
(J)	**Reduction in CO_2e per m^2**	**$kgCO_2e/m^2$**	$= I/10,000$	**0.6**	**9**
(K)	Total CO_2 emissions (base case)	$kgCO_2e/m^2$	Table 7.1	105	105
	% reduction		$= J/K$	0.6%	8.6%

Table 7.3 Maximum CO_2e reduction and sizing calculations of solar thermal in Building X and Hotel Y

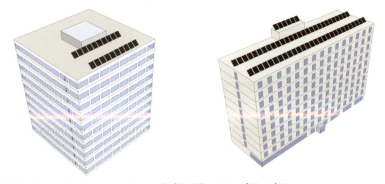

Fig 7.3 Solar thermal panels on the roof of Building X and Hotel Y

In office buildings solar thermal systems will reduce CO_2e emissions by less than 1%. In hotels it is possible for solar thermal to provide a 9% reduction. However, the calculation reveals a small problem with Hotel Y – there isn't enough room to fit all the panels on the 1,000 m^2 roof! The calculation was based on panels at a 60° tilt and this would require 2 m long panels to be spaced 6.5 m apart to reduce overshadowing in winter (refer to Appendix I for the spacing calculation). The solar panel to roof area ratio for panels at 60° in London is 27%, and assuming that 75% of the roof area is available for panels (some space is required for other roof plant) then the solar panel area is limited to 200 m^2. The CO_2e reduction from this reduced panel area on Hotel Y is $9.0 \times 200/969 =$ **1.9 $kgCO_2e/m^2$** (2% of total emissions). Figure 7.3 shows the panels on both buildings.

Detailed analysis of daily solar irradiation, tilt, panel spacing, thermal demands and storage is required to optimise the design to suit a particular building, including consideration of physical constraints and space requirements.

		Unit	Calculation	Building X	Hotel Y
(D)	Area of panel			65 m²	200 m²
(L)	Capital cost	£	= D × £500	£32,000	£100,000
(M)	Energy cost saving	£/year	= H × 3.5p	£1,050	£3,250
	Simple payback	Years	= M/L	30	31
(N)	Net present cost (15 yrs @ 5%)		Appendix I	£18,800	£59,200
	Cost per tCO$_2$e saved in 15 years	**£/tCO2e: 15 years @ 5%**	= (N × 15)/ (I × 1000)	**£210**	**£210**

Table 7.4 **Financial evaluation of solar thermal systems on Building X and Hotel Y**

Table 7.4 shows the simple financial payback for the solar thermal systems, assuming a capital cost based on £500 per m² of panel. The net present cost (NPC) is also shown for a 15-year period with an annual discount rate of 5% together with the cost per tonne of CO$_2$e saved over the same period. If the buildings did not have access to natural gas, and used LPG, heating oil or direct electricity (e.g. immersion heater) instead to generate domestic hot water, then the energy cost and CO$_2$e savings due to solar thermal would be significantly improved.

7.4 BIOMASS BOILERS

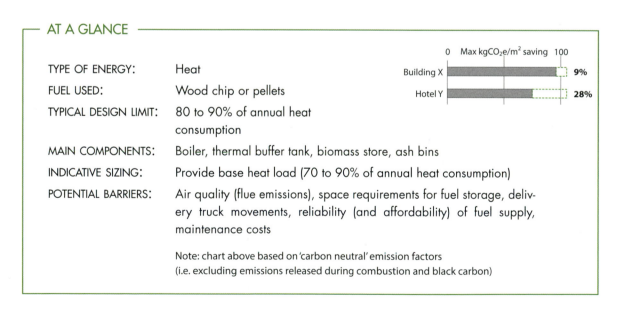

Biomass typically means biological material derived from living or recently living organisms. This can be converted into energy using a variety of different processes:

- heat energy through combustion, gasification and pyrolysis
- chemical energy through anaerobic digestion (methane) or fermentation (biofuel).

In commercial buildings the most common forms of biomass are wood pellet, wood chip and biofuels. Wood pellets are generally made from compacted sawdust to defined standards to ensure consistent calorific value, structure, density and moisture content.[10] Wood chips are more variable but are usually supplied with a moisture content of around 30%. Biofuels are discussed later in section 7.8 on CHP.

Figure 7.4 shows a typical biomass boiler arrangement. In theory, biomass could provide all of a building's heating demand; however, biomass boilers work best at constant load and so are often designed to provide between 70 and 90% of total annual demand with back-up gas boilers providing the remaining heat during peak periods (cold winter days) and periods of very low demand (summer). Biomass boilers can't ramp up and down as quickly as gas boilers to meet sudden spikes in demand and so thermal storage (buffer) tanks are installed to allow the boilers to run at constant loads.

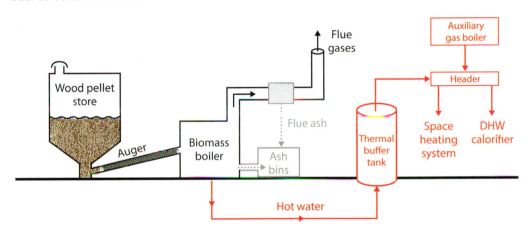

Fig 7.4 Typical biomass boiler configuration with natural gas auxiliary boilers

Wood chips have a lower fuel cost than wood pellets but also have a lower calorific value and bulk density.[11] This means that wood chips require around 3.5 times more storage volume than wood pellets for the same energy content, and consequently require more deliveries to site and larger storage tanks/hoppers. Wood pellets are therefore more suited to commercial buildings in urban environments as they require less storage space, have a consistent size, and produce less ash and particulate emissions. They also flow more like a liquid, allowing for automated boiler feeds and pumped deliveries from tankers.

The successful design of a biomass system must consider:

- size and control of biomass boilers to optimise efficient operation
- storage volume and proximity to plant room
- frequency and size of truck deliveries
- vehicle access to the building
- method of delivery – pumped, tipper truck/trailer or roll-on/roll-off.

Biomass boilers in Building X and Hotel Y

Table 7.5 provides a summary of the CO_2e savings, storage and delivery requirements for Building X and Hotel Y using a combination of wood pellet boilers and natural gas boilers. The assumptions and calculations are given in Appendix I. The contribution to global warming of black carbon and the time lag for new trees to reabsorb the CO_2 released from biomass combustion has not been included.[12]

Table 7.6 shows a simplified financial evaluation which includes the capital cost of the biomass system and the additional floor area required. As wood pellets are more expensive than natural gas, there is no financial payback with wood pellet boilers. However, no payback does not mean that biomass is the most costly method of reducing CO_2e, represented here by the $£/tCO_2e$ value.

	Unit	Building X	Hotel Y
% of annual heat energy from biomass		75%	85%
Reduction in CO_2e	**$kgCO_2e/m^2$**	**9**	**30**
% reduction in CO_2e		8%	28%
Volume of pellets for peak heating period	m^3/week	10	29
Wood pellet storage volume	m^3	32	50
Peak frequency of fuel deliveries	days	15	5

Table 7.5 Maximum CO_2e reduction and wood pellet storage requirements of biomass boilers in Building X and Hotel Y

	Unit	Building X	Hotel Y
Capital cost	£	£245,000	£350,000
Energy cost increase	£/year	£7,760	£25,780
Simple payback	years	none	none
Net present cost (15 years @ 7.5%)		£342,200	£673,000
Cost per tCO_2e saved over 15 years	**$£/tCO_2e$: 15 years @ 5%**	**£260**	**£150**

Table 7.6 Financial evaluation of biomass boilers in Building X and Hotel Y

Wood chips are typically cheaper than natural gas (<2.5p/kWh) but there are issues with delivery truck frequency and storage requirements. Consequently, wood chips are not suited to most city centre buildings.

The financial evaluation has excluded the maintenance costs associated with removing ash bins, cleaning the boilers and keeping the mechanical auger fuel supply systems working smoothly. These costs are higher for wood chips due to the higher variability in fuel quality compared to wood pellets.

If the biomass storage is located at ground floor level then this may take up valuable floor space which could otherwise be rented for offices or retail. Annual city centre rentals in the UK can vary from £100/m^2 to over £500/m^2 so this could also influence the financial feasibility of using biomass.

AREA OF PLANTATION REQUIRED

Short rotation coppice (SRC) willow plantations in the UK can provide 46 MWh of biomass energy annually per hectare.[13] If this is converted into wood pellets to supply biomass boilers (replacing natural gas boilers) then the carbon saving is 6.8 tCO_2e per hectare. Figure 7.5 shows the area of such plantation required to provide fuel to the biomass boilers in Building X and Hotel Y.

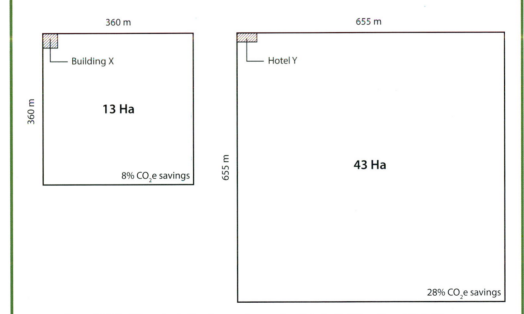

Fig 7.5 Area of SRC willow plantation to supply wood pellets to Building X and Hotel Y

7.5 HEAT PUMPS

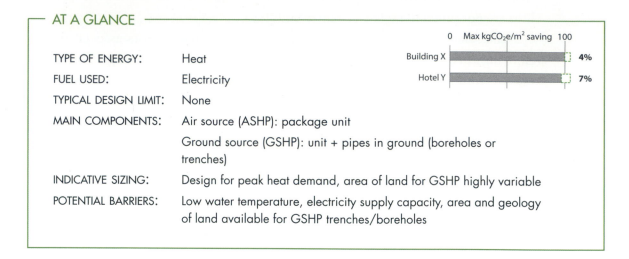

		0 Max kgCO₂e/m² saving 100
TYPE OF ENERGY:	Heat	Building X — 4%
FUEL USED:	Electricity	Hotel Y — 7%
TYPICAL DESIGN LIMIT:	None	
MAIN COMPONENTS:	Air source (ASHP): package unit	
	Ground source (GSHP): unit + pipes in ground (boreholes or trenches)	
INDICATIVE SIZING:	Design for peak heat demand, area of land for GSHP highly variable	
POTENTIAL BARRIERS:	Low water temperature, electricity supply capacity, area and geology of land available for GSHP trenches/boreholes	

A heat pump is an electrical device that uses the refrigeration cycle to extract heat from one place and transfer it to another (refer to Figure 7.6). It can provide either heating or cooling depending on which way the refrigerant flows around the system. Every home has a type of heat pump – a fridge pumps heat from the food (making it cold) and moves it to the back of the fridge (which gets warm).

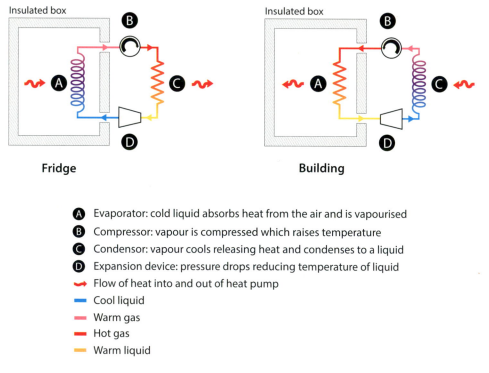

A Evaporator: cold liquid absorbs heat from the air and is vapourised
B Compressor: vapour is compressed which raises temperature
C Condenser: vapour cools releasing heat and condenses to a liquid
D Expansion device: pressure drops reducing temperature of liquid
➝ Flow of heat into and out of heat pump
▬ Cool liquid
▬ Warm gas
▬ Hot gas
▬ Warm liquid

Fig 7.6 The basic components and refrigerant flows in a heat pump

A heat pump provides an efficient way of turning electricity into heat. The efficiency with which it does this is expressed as the coefficient of performance (CoP), which is the ratio of heat energy out to electrical energy in.

CoP = heat energy output/heat energy input

For example, a CoP of 3 delivers 3 kWh of heat for every 1 kWh of electrical energy input. In comparison, an electric bar heater would have a CoP of around 1. The CoP varies with the temperature difference between the evaporator (heat source) and the condenser (heat supplied) – the larger the difference, the lower the CoP.[14] Consequently, heat pumps are typically not used to supply domestic hot water when natural gas is available because delivering water temperatures of 60 °C significantly reduces the efficiency.

The classification of heat pumps as renewable energy is contentious. A heat pump with a CoP less than 2.7 has higher CO_2e emissions than an efficient natural gas boiler in the UK. The EU and the UK Government have set various, often inconsistent, criteria for the minimum CoP of heat pumps to be classed as renewable. This is discussed further in Appendix I.

Gas Absorption Heat Pumps (GAHP), which use a natural gas burner to drive the refrigeration cycle instead of a compressor driven by an electric motor, deliver around 1.5 kWh of heat for every 1 kWh of natural gas input. They consequently have lower carbon emissions and energy costs than electric heat pumps in the UK and are discussed further in Appendix I.

Types of heat pump

Heat pumps come in a variety of configurations based on what the evaporator (heat source) and condenser (heat delivery) are connected to. Figure 7.7 (overleaf) summarises the four main options. 'Ground source' uses water in pipes to transfer heat from the ground, aquifers or water bodies to the heat pump condenser.

Ground source heat pumps (GSHP) are usually more efficient than air source heat pumps (ASHP) because they pump heat from the ground, which typically contains more heat energy (i.e. it's warmer) than air in the winter. But they have an additional capital cost due to the network of horizontal or vertical pipes installed in the ground, the extent of which is dependent on the type of ground and area of land available. If the system is undersized then the ground can freeze (and swell) if too much heat is pumped out of it. Aquifers and large, stable water bodies (sea, rivers, lakes) can also be used as a heat source.

Heat pumps can provide all of the space heating demand in buildings. However, simply connecting a heat pump to an existing gas boiler heating system will not give

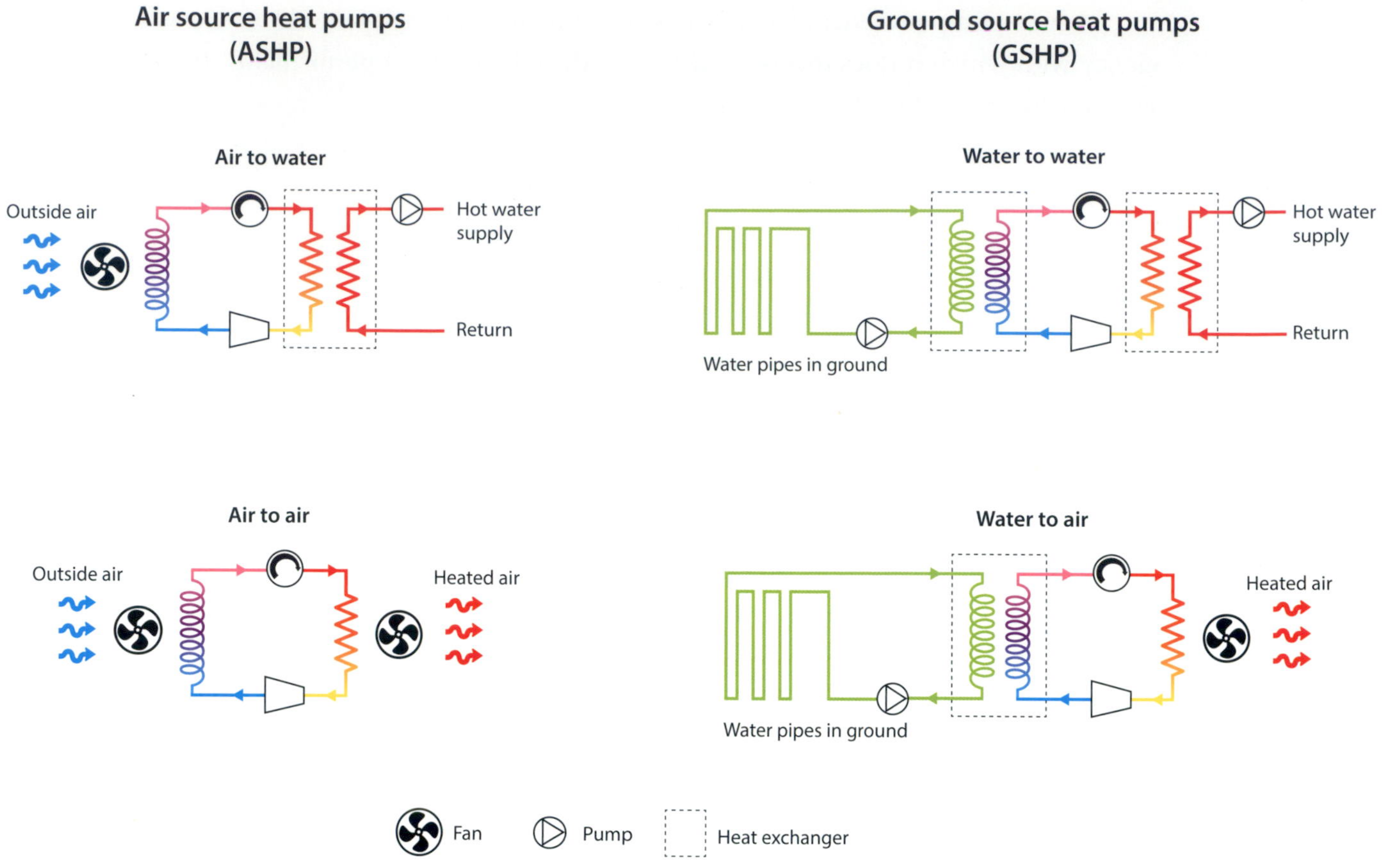

Air source heat pumps (ASHP)

Ground source heat pumps (GSHP)

Air to water

Outside air

Hot water supply

Return

Water to water

Hot water supply

Return

Water pipes in ground

Air to air

Outside air

Heated air

Water to air

Heated air

Water pipes in ground

Fan   Pump   Heat exchanger

Fig 7.7 Typical heat pump configurations

out enough heat. This is because most heat pumps provide a lower temperature of hot water (typically between 35 and 45 °C) compared to gas boilers (up to 80 °C) and so larger radiators or coils are needed in the building heating system to distribute the heat into the space.

Variable refrigerant flow (VRF) systems are commonly used in new commercial buildings as they provide both heating and cooling, replacing the separate gas boiler and electric chiller systems, but they do not necessarily deliver any net CO_2e savings.[15] VRF systems are typically air to air or water to air heat pumps, with refrigerant pipes replacing the heating and chilled water pipes to the fan coil units throughout the building. The power supply can be connected directly to a tenant's electricity meter, which simplifies billing arrangements.

How do heat pumps perform in operation?

In theory, ASHPs should have an annual average CoP of at least 3 and GSHPs a CoP of 4, but this is not always achieved in practice. The measured CoP of domestic heat

	Worst CoP	Average CoP	Best CoP	Typical stated CoP
Air source	1.2	2.2	3.3	3 to 4
Ground source	1.3	2.4	3.6	4 to 5

Table 7.7 Summary of UK domestic heat pump trials by Energy Savings Trust in 2010

pumps in the UK during a field trial[16] in 2010 were typically much lower than many suppliers/installers state (refer to Table 7.7). Very few installations outperformed a 90% efficient natural gas boiler. The difference between air source and ground source heat pumps in the trial was surprisingly small – particularly given the additional expense.

The results of the trial do not necessarily mean that heat pump installations will always perform this poorly. Other trials in Europe and Japan suggest that CoPs of around 3 should be achievable for ASHP and typically between 3.5 and 4 for GSHP.[17] Good design, installation and controls are clearly important to turn theoretical performance into reality.

To give purchasers a more realistic prediction of likely performance, the EU has introduced the Seasonal Coefficient of Performance (SCoP), which together with estimated annual energy consumption, must be stated on the Energy Efficiency Labels of heat pumps under 12kW from January 2013.[18] It takes into account how a system performs at different temperatures during a heating season in three different climate zones, instead of its efficiency at a fixed test temperature of 7 °C.

HEAT PUMPS IN AIR HANDLING UNITS

As stated previously, heat pumps work most efficiently with low temperature differences between the heat source and the heat emitter. Figure 7.8 (overleaf) shows the integration of an ASHP into an air handling unit (AHU) to temper the fresh air supply in a building. The external unit (evaporator and fan) normally located on the roof is replaced by coils in the exhaust air stream. The ASHP is effectively acting as a second heat recovery system.

Since the exhaust air stream is warmer than the outside air, the heat pump works more efficiently. By only tempering the fresh air supply, the heating coils (condenser) in the AHU are at a low temperature and, consequently, the temperature difference between evaporator and condenser is less than 25 °C on a cold winter day. This means the CoP will be between 5 and 6, which is much better than a typical ASHP. On milder days the CoP could rise to 9, with an average for the year of 7 to 8.

continued overleaf

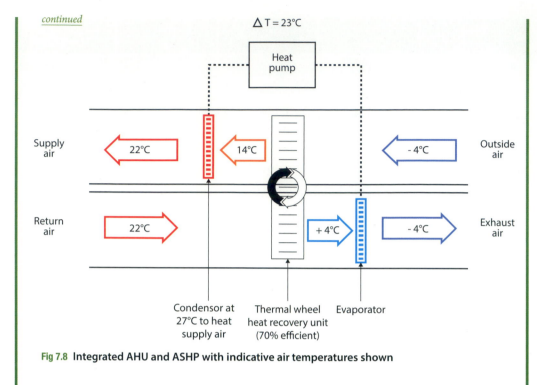

Fig 7.8 **Integrated AHU and ASHP with indicative air temperatures shown**

Some issues to note:

- The AHU heat pump is not heating the whole building, only the fresh air supply. Space heating and cooling (radiators, fan coil units, chilled beams, etc.) is still required to deal with heat losses through the building fabric.
- The fan energy in the AHU will increase due to locating the evaporator in the exhaust air duct and this needs to be considered when calculating the overall system efficiency.
- The system can operate in reverse to provide tempered (cool) supply air in the summer.

Heat pumps in Building X and Hotel Y

Figure 7.9 shows the CO_2e savings for different heat pump CoPs compared to a natural gas boiler assuming that heat pumps provide all space heating (but not domestic hot water) in Building X and Hotel Y. A ground source heat pump with a CoP of 4 would reduce Building X's emissions by **5 kgCO$_2$e/m^2** (4%) and Hotel Y's by **10 kgCO$_2$e/m^2** (9%).

If 200 m deep closed loop boreholes, spaced at 6 m centres, were used then the area of land required would be 2,160 m^2 in Building X and 2,700 m^2 in Hotel Y. This is greater than the footprint of both buildings (1,000 m^2). If the land area for boreholes

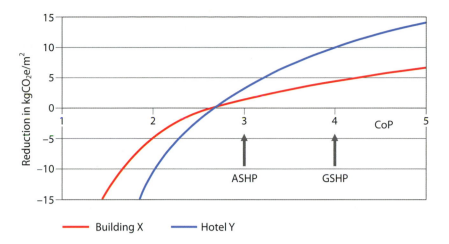

Fig 7.9 Annual CO_2e reductions for space heating heat pumps in Building X and Hotel Y

was limited to 1,000 m² then 36 boreholes could be installed. This limits the amount of heat that can be extracted from the ground and alternative heat sources would be required during peak heating periods.

Table 7.8 summarises the calculations in Appendix I for three heat pump scenarios:

- ASHPs only
- GSHPs only
- combination of GSHPs (with 36 boreholes) and ASHP.

	Building X			Hotel Y		
	ASHP	Both	GSHP	ASHP	Both	GSHP
Heat pump CoP (annual average)	2.8	3.8	4	2.8	3.6	4
kgCO₂e saving	5,000	40,526	45,500	10,714	75,000	97,500
kgCO₂e/m² saving per year	**0.5**	**4.1**	**4.6**	**1.1**	**7.5**	**9.8**
Energy cost saving per year	£2,000	£7,921	£8,750	£4,286	£15,000	£18,750
Length of boreholes (m)	0	7,200	12,000	0	7,200	12,000
Cost (@ £50 per m of borehole)	£0	£360,000	£600,000	£0	£360,000	£600,000
Payback period (years)	**0**	**45**	**69**	**0**	**24**	**32**
Net present cost (15 years @ 5%)		£260,750	£490,370		£172,050	£365,070
£/tCO₂e: 15 years @ 5%		**£430**	**£720**		**£155**	**£250**

Table 7.8 Maximum CO_2e reduction and cost/benefit of ASHPs and GSHPs in Building X and Hotel Y

For the cost benefit analysis, ASHPs are assumed to cost the same as the base case building's heating and cooling system. The capital cost is actually lower but they need to be replaced after 10 to 12 years, which gives a life cycle cost at 15 years similar to traditional systems. The additional cost of GSHPs is primarily due to the capital cost of the boreholes, assumed to be £50/m.

GSHPs provide relatively small CO_2e and energy cost savings compared to ASHPs, so unless the ground system can be installed relatively cheaply, or the building owner wishes to avoid all the condenser units sitting on the roof (or, even worse, hanging off the façade of the building) for aesthetic reasons, it is usually difficult to justify the additional capital cost.

The combined ground and air source option with 36 boreholes provides almost the same CO_2e and energy savings as a full ground source system, but is a more economically viable solution. This is because the GSHP is assumed to be providing around 85% of the annual heating consumption in Building X (70% in Hotel Y), with the less efficient ASHP only kicking in during peak heating periods.

The calculations of borehole length are indicative only. Detailed geological testing and modelling are necessary to determine the heat transfer between the ground and the boreholes and the thermal capacity of the ground. They also do not take into account any potential reduction in total borehole length if the heat pumps are also used for cooling and reject heat into the ground in summer, which can later be extracted in the winter. The geological analysis of heat transfer and heat capacity of the ground can become quite complex.

Finally, the calculations do not consider greenhouse gas emissions due to F-gases (refrigerants) leaking to the atmosphere. In Building X this could be around **1 to 2 kgCO$_2$e/m^2 per annum** (refer to Appendix B), which would reduce the carbon reduction benefit of heat pumps used for heating.

The future for heat pumps

To meet international greenhouse gas reduction targets, most countries will seek to reduce the carbon content of grid electricity by increasing the amount of electricity generated by renewable sources (e.g. wind and solar farms) and low carbon sources (e.g. nuclear). Heat pumps will therefore increasingly become a more attractive source of heating based on:

- lower GHG emissions
- security of supply – electricity can be generated from a variety of sources
- energy costs – as gas reserves reduce (or become harder to extract) then the cost of natural gas will rise.

WHAT IS THE BEST WAY TO USE NATURAL GAS TO GENERATE HEAT?

Natural gas can be used to generate grid electricity in gas turbine power stations or it can be used to produce heat directly in buildings. Since natural gas is a finite resource (the UK is now a net importer of gas) what is the most efficient use of this resource to provide heating in buildings? Figure 7.10 considers 100 kWh of natural gas and shows how much heat is delivered to a building using three options:

- converting the gas into electricity in new 55% efficient combined cycle gas turbine (CCGT) power stations[19] and then using ASHPs in buildings to generate heat
- using gas absorption heat pumps
- using gas boilers in buildings.

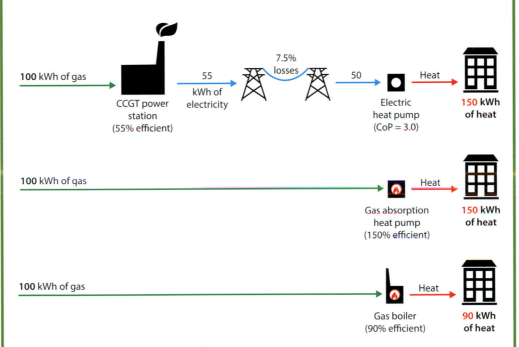

Fig 7.10 Using natural gas to heat buildings

From this simple exercise it appears that using gas to generate electricity in new, efficient CCGT power stations and then using heat pumps to provide space heating in buildings is a more energy and carbon efficient solution than gas boilers, provided that the heat pump has an annual average CoP greater than 1.8. Gas absorption heat pumps have a similar net gas efficiency to using CCGT and ASHPs.

7.6 PHOTOVOLTAICS

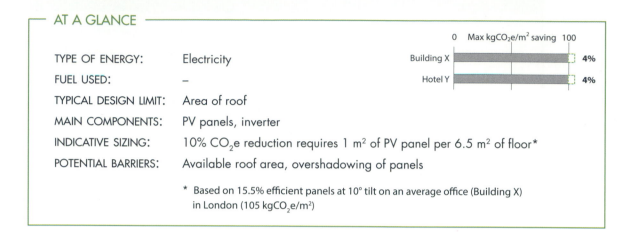

AT A GLANCE

TYPE OF ENERGY:	Electricity
FUEL USED:	–
TYPICAL DESIGN LIMIT:	Area of roof
MAIN COMPONENTS:	PV panels, inverter
INDICATIVE SIZING:	10% CO_2e reduction requires 1 m² of PV panel per 6.5 m² of floor*
POTENTIAL BARRIERS:	Available roof area, overshadowing of panels

* Based on 15.5% efficient panels at 10° tilt on an average office (Building X) in London (105 $kgCO_2e$/m²)

Photovoltaic (PV) solar panels convert solar energy directly into low voltage direct current (DC) electricity (typically between 12 and 24V).[20] An inverter converts this to alternating current (AC) at a voltage to match the mains electricity supply so that it can be connected to the building's electrical distribution system. Surplus electricity can be fed back into the grid (refer to Figure 7.11).

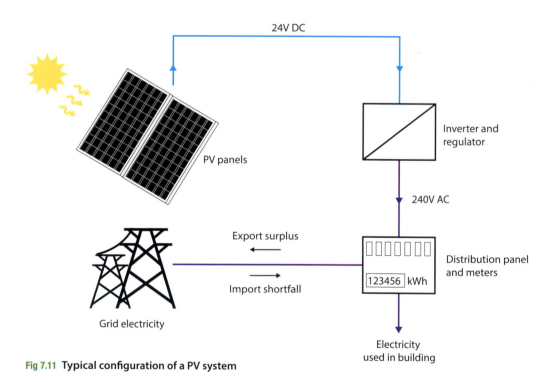

Fig 7.11 Typical configuration of a PV system

The amount of electricity generated by a PV panel depends on the amount of solar energy hitting the panel, and the efficiency with which this is converted into electricity. The solar energy, called the solar irradiation, is typically expressed in kWh/m² per annum, and varies with:

- location – it is sunnier in the Sahara than it is in England
- orientation – which influences how many hours the panel receives direct sunlight
- tilt – which influences the angle at which the sun's rays strike the panel
- overshadowing – how often the panel is in shade (from trees, buildings and other panels).

Appendix I provides some typical values for solar irradiation in the UK and guidelines for panel spacing to reduce overshadowing.

A range of photovoltaic products is available, with varying costs and efficiencies.[21] The most commonly used on buildings are shown in Table 7.9.

	Hybrid panels	Monocrystalline	Polycrystalline	Thin film
Typical module efficiency	Up to 20%	12–16%	10–13%	3–6%
Cost per m²	Highest		⟶	Lowest

Table 7.9 Typical PV panel types used on buildings

As a technology, photovoltaics are very simple to include in buildings – put a few panels on the roof, connect the wires to an inverter and wait for the sun to shine. Figure 7.12 shows the most common methods of placing PV panels on buildings. PV cells can also be incorporated into glazing panels and the development of new PV technologies will open up further possibilities.

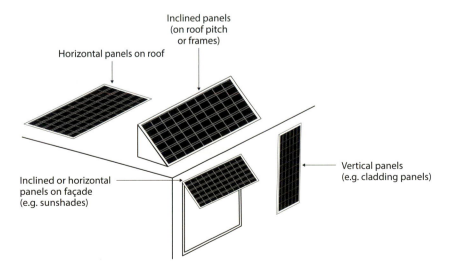

Fig 7.12 Typical applications of PV on buildings

Estimating the energy generated and CO_2 reduction

The maximum electricity that can be generated by PV panels on Building X is calculated based on the following assumptions:

- 300 m² of PV panels are installed on the roof facing south at 10° tilt (reduction in output from overshadowing from the plant room has been ignored)
- 320 m² of PV panel sunshades are installed on the south façade at 30° tilt
- the grid infrastructure (and utility company) will allow surplus electricity generated by PV to be exported from the building
- the roof and south façade of the building are not overshadowed by adjacent buildings.

Figure 7.13 shows how the panels would look on Building X.

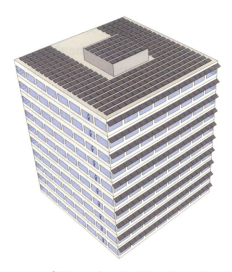

Fig 7.13 Arrangement of PV panels on Building X to deliver 5% CO_2e reduction

The capital cost per kW varies depending on the size of the system.[23] The capital cost of Building X's PV system is based on £1,500/kW for a 120 kW system. Table 7.11 shows the CO_2e reductions and cost/benefit due to the PV system on Building X. The results for Hotel Y are assumed to be similar. If the UK's PV feed-in tariffs were applied in 2013, the payback reduces to under 10 years.[24]

	Unit	Roof	Sunshades	Total
Annual solar irradiation	kWh/m2	1,048	1,141	
Area of panels	**m²**	**300**	**320**	**620**
System capacity	kW	47	50	96
Solar energy on panels	kWh	314,559	365,249	679,808
PV system efficiency		11.1%		
Electricity generated	kWh	35,003	40,644	75,647
CO_2e reduction per annum	$kgCO_2$e	21,002	24,386	45,388
CO_2e reduction per annum	**$kgCO_2/m^2$**	**2.1**	**2.4**	**4.5**
Capital cost	(£1,500/kW)	£69,770	£74,400	£144,170
Energy cost saving per annum	(£0.10/kWh)	£3,500	£4,064	£7,565
Payback	Years	20	18	19
Net present cost (15 years @ 5%)				£49,387
£/tCO_2e: 15 years @ 5%				**£73**

Table 7.11 Maximum CO_2e reduction and cost/benefit of photovoltaic panels on Building X

ZERO CARBON USING PHOTOVOLTAICS?

To make Building X 'zero carbon' using photovoltaics alone would require 1,750 MWh of electricity to be generated to offset the total building emissions (gas and electricity) of 105 $kgCO_2e/m^2$. The required area of monocrystalline PV panels at 10° tilt is 15,000 m^2 which equates to 1.5 m^2 of panel area for every 1 m^2 of floor. Figure 7.14 shows the area of roof needed (24,500 m^2). The capital cost of the 2.3 MWe system (excluding the roof) would be around £2.3 million (£230/m^2 of GIA).

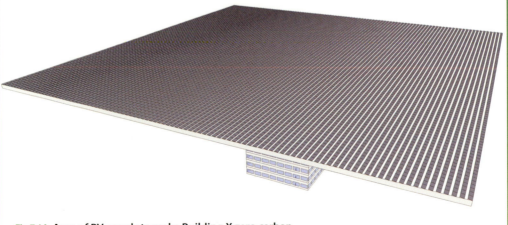

Fig 7.14 Area of PV panels to make Building X zero carbon

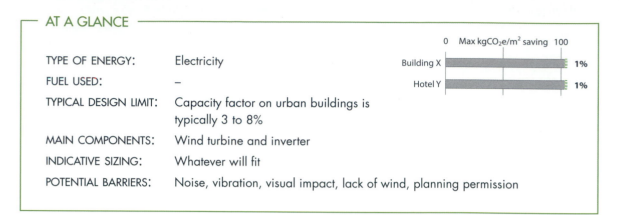

7.7 WIND TURBINES

AT A GLANCE

TYPE OF ENERGY:	Electricity
FUEL USED:	–
TYPICAL DESIGN LIMIT:	Capacity factor on urban buildings is typically 3 to 8%
MAIN COMPONENTS:	Wind turbine and inverter
INDICATIVE SIZING:	Whatever will fit
POTENTIAL BARRIERS:	Noise, vibration, visual impact, lack of wind, planning permission

A wind turbine converts wind energy into rotary motion to drive a generator to produce electricity. Before considering how wind turbines can be used on buildings it is first necessary to understand how much power is available from wind in different locations.

Getting power from wind

The power available from wind is a function of the cube of the wind speed, so doubling the wind speed increases the power by eight times. Clearly, the best place to put wind turbines is where it is windy! Now consider commercial onshore and offshore wind farms and you'll notice two things:

1 The turbines are horizontal axis with diameters between 40 and 80 m, sitting atop big masts placing them 50 to 100 m above ground level.
2 There is a dearth of buildings underneath them.

Any obstructions near ground level, such as trees and buildings, create drag which reduces wind speed. This is why wind turbines are placed as far away from the ground and other obstructions as possible. Figure 7.15 illustrates the typical difference in wind speeds between urban turbines and wind farms.

A typical 12 kWe wind turbine (the 'e' stands for electricity) produces 12 kW of electricity only when the rated wind speed is reached (typically around 10 to 12m/s). Wind speeds above this do not generate more power – the turbine is already running at its maximum capacity. However, for much of the year, the wind speed will be below this, and the electricity generated is therefore less. On calm days the turbines will not rotate at all until the cut-in speed is reached (typically between 1.5 and 3.5 m/s).

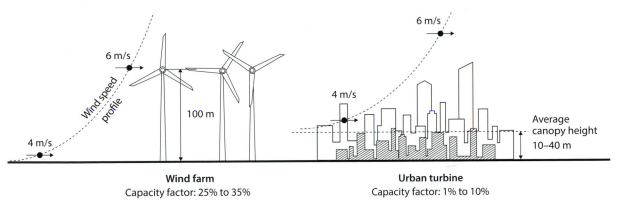

Wind farm
Capacity factor: 25% to 35%

Urban turbine
Capacity factor: 1% to 10%

Fig 7.15 **Typical wind speeds and capacity factors for urban and rural wind turbines**

To predict the annual electricity from wind turbines requires detailed calculations using wind speed distributions at the particular site (the number of hours each wind speed occurs during the year) and the turbine power curve (how much electricity is generated at each wind speed). Fortunately, there is a quick ballpark method of estimating the annual electricity for feasibility purposes without having to perform detailed analysis. The capacity factor is the ratio of electricity generated in a year compared to the maximum possible output from a wind turbine.

$$\text{capacity factor (\%)} = \frac{\text{annual electricity generated (kWh)}}{\text{turbine capacity (kW)} \times 365 \text{ days} \times 24 \text{ hours}}$$

So, if the likely capacity factor for a site is known, then a rough estimate of how much electricity might be generated is given by:

$$\text{annual electricity (kWh/annum)} = \text{turbine capacity (kWe)} \times \text{capacity factor (\%)} \times 8{,}760 \text{ hours}$$

This is not an accurate calculation, but does provide a useful sanity check as to whether it is worth pursuing a wind turbine option on a particular site or building.

A capacity factor of 10% is often assumed for building-mounted turbines in the UK but this is rarely achieved in practice. Various wind trials suggest a value of between 1 and 8% for urban wind turbines.[25] In comparison, the average capacity factor for commercial wind farms in the UK in 2011 was 30% (with 27% for onshore and 37% for offshore).[26]

Assuming an urban capacity factor of 5%, a 10 kWe wind turbine on a city centre building generates 4,380 kWh/annum (10 kW × 5% × 8,760 hours). If the same turbine was located on top of a windy hill in Scotland (with a 30% capacity factor) it would generate six times the amount of electricity.

Types of wind turbine

Figure 7.16 shows the two basic types of wind turbine, horizontal axis (HAWT) and vertical axis (VAWT). These come in different shapes and sizes. Wind farms rarely use vertical axis turbines – and for a good reason – they are not as efficient or cost effective as horizontal axis turbines. They do have a few advantages in urban settings: they look funkier, don't need to be mounted as high above buildings and are claimed to respond better to variable wind directions and turbulence (such as found at the top of buildings).

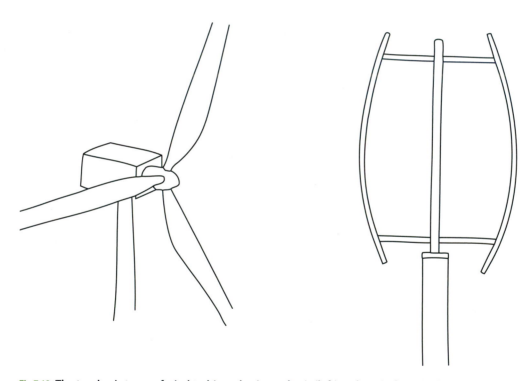

Fig 7.16 **The two basic types of wind turbine – horizontal axis (left) and vertical axis (right)**

Putting wind turbines on buildings

Urban wind turbines are usually put on poles on the top of a building – the higher the better to experience higher wind speeds and to avoid the turbulent air zone that occurs around the top of buildings. As a rule of thumb, the turbine should be at least 10 m above the highest surface of the building (or adjacent buildings if these are taller). To reduce wake losses and turbulence (due to an upwind turbine disrupting wind on downstream turbines) it is recommended to have a minimum spacing of 5× rotor diameter between turbines.

It is difficult to make turbines on poles visually appealing and so obtaining planning permission may not be straightforward. In addition to aesthetics, other potential barriers include height restrictions, light flicker, noise and vibration. A number of buildings have attempted to integrate the turbines into the fabric of the building, and this requires even more careful consideration of turbulent air flows around the building.

However, before getting to this stage in the design and planning process, the key question is: can wind turbines make a meaningful contribution to reducing the CO_2e emissions of city centre commercial buildings?

Wind turbines on Building X

Table 7.12 (overleaf) shows the contribution that wind turbines can make on Building X. These are relatively small (1 to 2%) despite some generous assumptions with the capacity factors (which, in reality, could be half these in some city centre locations). The cost per tCO_2e saved is over £650.

Clearly, bigger wind turbines are needed to make a serious dent on Building X's carbon footprint. Putting aside issues with planning, aesthetics, noise, vibration and common sense, Figure 7.17 shows the CO_2e savings from 6 m, 27 m and 54 m diameter turbines on the roof of Building X compared to if they were located on a remote windy hill.[27] The conclusion is fairly obvious – city centres are not the best location for wind farms!

To make Building X carbon neutral would require 670 kWe of wind turbine capacity to be located at a site with a capacity factor of 30%. This would have a capital cost of approximately £1 million which is £100/m² of GIA (compared to PVs which would cost £230/m² of GIA).

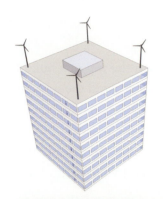
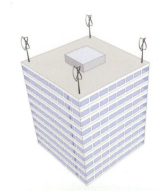
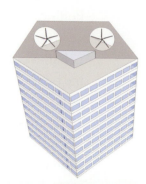

	1 Horizontal axis	2 Vertical axis	3 Building integrated
Turbine capacity	6 kW	12 kW	19 kW
Number of turbines	4	4	2
Total capacity	24 kW	48 kW	38 kW
Capacity factor	8%	8%	5%
Annual output	16,820 kWh	33,640 kWh	16,640 kWh
CO_2 reduction	10,090 kgCO$_2$e	20,180 kgCO$_2$e	9,990 kgCO$_2$e
Reduction in CO$_2$e (kgCO$_2$e/m²)	1	2	1
% reduction	1%	2%	1%
Cost per kW[28]	£5,000	£7,000	£13,000
Capital cost	£120,000	£336,000	£495,000
Annual cost saving*	£1,680	£3,360	£1,660
Simple payback	71 years	100 years	300 years
Net present cost	£98,925	£293,850	£473,150
£/tCO$_2$e: 15 years @ 5%	**£655**	**£970**	**£3,160**

* The wind also blows in off-peak periods when the cost of electricity is less than the peak tariff.

The analysis above ignores this – which makes the financial evaluation here more favourable than it actually is.

Table 7.12   Maximum CO$_2$e reduction and cost/benefit of wind turbines on Building X

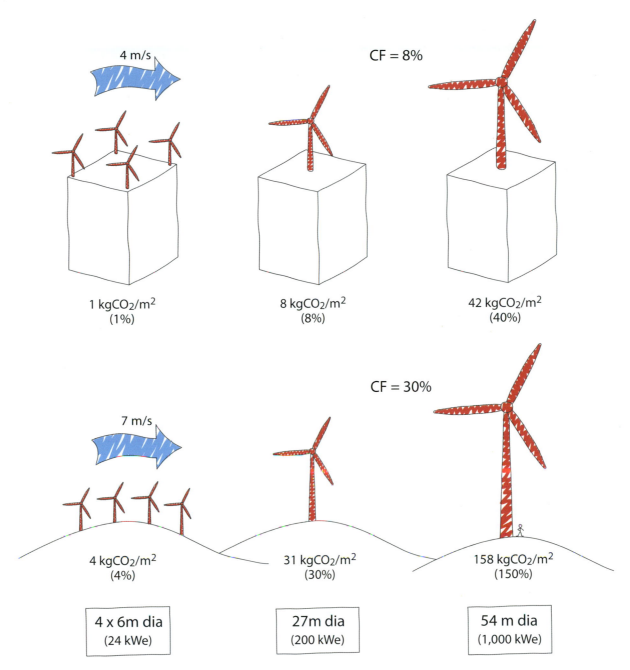

4 m/s

CF = 8%

1 kgCO$_2$/m^2
(1%)

8 kgCO$_2$/m^2
(8%)

42 kgCO$_2$/m^2
(40%)

CF = 30%

7 m/s

4 kgCO$_2$/m^2
(4%)

31 kgCO$_2$/m^2
(30%)

158 kgCO$_2$/m^2
(150%)

4 x 6m dia
(24 kWe)

27m dia
(200 kWe)

54 m dia
(1,000 kWe)

Fig 7.17 Comparison of outputs from 6 m, 27 m and 52 m diameter turbines
on Building X and on a windy hill (expressed as the reduction in Building X's carbon footprint)

IS IT WORTH BOTHERING WITH BUILDING MOUNTED WIND TURBINES?

The typical capital cost for a turbine in a large scale wind farm (100 MW to 300 MW) is between £1,000 and £2,800 per kW of installed capacity.[29] Assuming a cost of £1,500 per kW, Table 7.13 shows how the life cycle costs compare to a building mounted turbine at £5,000 per kW.

	Wind farm	Building mounted
Capital cost per kW	£1,500	£5,000
Capacity factor	30%	8%
Annual electricity per installed kW	2,630 kWh	700 kWh
Annual CO_2 saved per installed kW	1,580 kgCO_2e	420 kgCO_2e
Electricity cost	6p/kWh*	10p/kWh
Annual electricity cost saving per kW	£158	£70
Simple payback**	10 years	71 years
£/tCO_2e: 15 years @ 5%	**-£20**	**£655**

* Assume 40% reduction for electricity distribution costs from turbine to building via national grid.

** Excludes any government incentives to generate renewable energy.

Table 7.13 **CO_2e and cost comparison between building turbines and wind farms**

The case is pretty compelling – electricity generation from a wind farm has capital costs less than half that of building mounted turbines, and delivers about four times the carbon savings. Instead of wasting money putting wind turbines on buildings to meet arbitrary on-site renewable energy targets, governments need to make it easy for building owners and developers to own, or part own, turbines in commercial wind farms.

Putting a wind turbine on an urban building is like putting a solar panel in permanent shade.

7.8 COMBINED HEAT AND POWER

AT A GLANCE

TYPE OF ENERGY: Heat and electricity

FUEL USED: Gas or biofuel

TYPICAL DESIGN LIMIT: Seasonal heat demand

MAIN COMPONENTS: Gas CHP: engine and generator

    Biofuel CHP: engine, generator and fuel storage tank

    Trigeneration: CHP plus absorption chiller

INDICATIVE SIZING: Provide annual base heating demand

POTENTIAL BARRIERS: Limited operating hours (<4,500/year), low annual heat to power energy consumption ratio, high peak heat to base heat energy demand, grid infrastructure

---

Combined heat and power (CHP) or cogeneration, uses fuel to generate electricity and heat for use in buildings. The amount of CO_2e emissions saved by using CHP depends on:

- the type and efficiency of the CHP unit
- how much of the heat generated is utilised in the building
- the carbon intensity of the grid electricity compared to the carbon intensity of the CHP fuel.

CHP type and efficiency

Table 7.14 (overleaf) shows four of the most common CHP systems to convert fuel energy into electricity and heat.[30]

Reciprocating engines (basically a petrol or diesel engine) are most suited to building applications where production of hot water, rather than steam, is the main requirement (refer to Figure 7.18). Their fast start-up times mean they could also form part of a building's emergency generator set. Fuel cells are also suitable in buildings.

Gas and biofuel can be used in building-based CHP systems. The most commonly used fuel in CHP is natural gas which is not a renewable energy source. Biomass (e.g. wood chip) and waste fuel sources tend to be used either in larger 'boiler and steam turbine' CHP systems or are converted into a synthetic gas to replace natural gas. These are more suited to industrial systems or district energy networks than individual buildings.

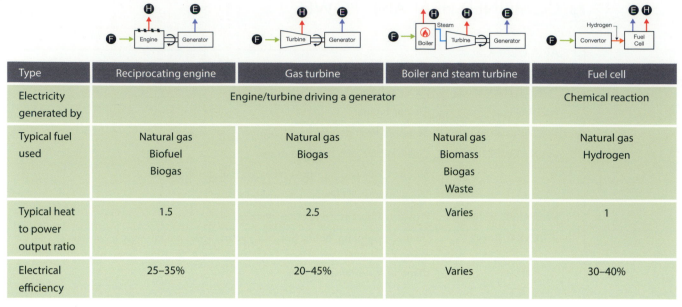

Type	Reciprocating engine	Gas turbine	Boiler and steam turbine	Fuel cell
Electricity generated by	Engine/turbine driving a generator			Chemical reaction
Typical fuel used	Natural gas Biofuel Biogas	Natural gas Biogas	Natural gas Biomass Biogas Waste	Natural gas Hydrogen
Typical heat to power output ratio	1.5	2.5	Varies	1
Electrical efficiency	25–35%	20–45%	Varies	30–40%

Table 7.14 **Main types of CHP systems**

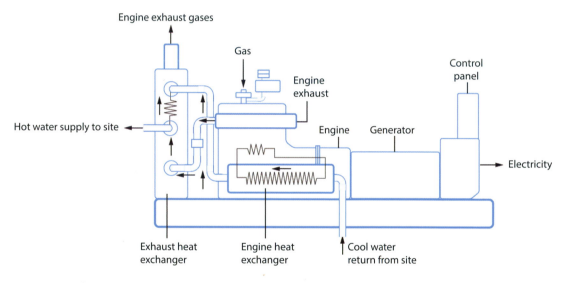

Fig 7.18 **Typical reciprocating engine package CHP plant used in buildings (source: The Carbon Trust)**

Gas CHP will be discussed first to illustrate how the use of CHP can reduce CO_2e emissions in buildings. The use of biofuel CHP is then considered.

The importance of using all of the heat

The effective use of heat is critical to making CHP viable. Figure 7.19 illustrates three scenarios for using the heat output from a typical natural gas reciprocating engine CHP in the UK:[31]

A **Trigeneration** – an absorption chiller (with a CoP of 0.7) is used to convert heat to chilled water, replacing that produced by an electric chiller (assumed to have a CoP of 5). When not used for cooling, the heat is used for heating. This system is sometimes known as combined cooling heating and power (CCHP).

B **Cogeneration** – the heat replaces that produced by a 90% efficient gas boiler. This is a conventional CHP system.

C **'One-generation'** – the heat is not used and is rejected, typically using an air-cooled heat rejection unit. The electrical fan energy used to dissipate the excess heat is assumed to be 0.15 kW for every kW of heat rejected.

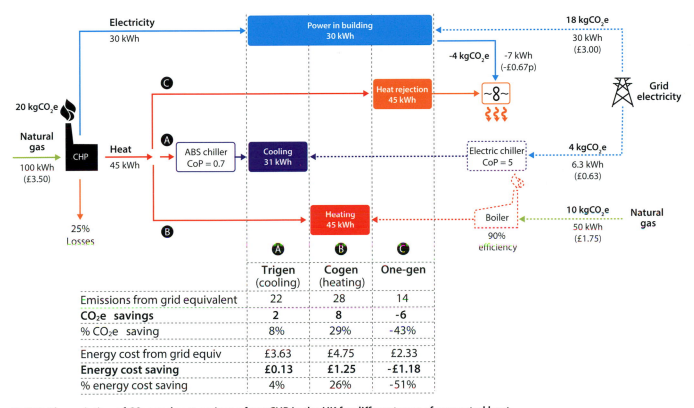

	A	B	C
	Trigen (cooling)	Cogen (heating)	One-gen
Emissions from grid equivalent	22	28	14
CO$_2$e savings	2	8	-6
% CO$_2$e saving	8%	29%	-43%
Energy cost from grid equiv	£3.63	£4.75	£2.33
Energy cost saving	£0.13	£1.25	-£1.18
% energy cost saving	4%	26%	-51%

Fig 7.19 The variation of CO$_2$e and cost savings of gas CHP in the UK for different uses of generated heat

This simple exercise is quite revealing. Based on the assumptions and efficiencies shown in Figure 7.19, acting as a 'one-generation' system (C), if all of the heat from the CHP is rejected then the net electricity output (30 – 7 = 23 kWh) is 43% more carbon intensive to produce (20 kgCO$_2$e) than obtaining it from the national grid (14 kgCO$_2$e). It is also 50% more expensive (£3.5 compared to £2.3). The carbon reduction benefit and financial viability of using CHP in the UK relies on the effective use of the heat output – wasting heat is a waste of money. In countries with more carbon intensive electricity grids, such as Australia, rejecting heat can still deliver a net CO$_2$e reduction, but it won't be cost effective.[32]

If all of the heat is used for heating purposes (B) then the net CO_2e emissions reduce by 29% (and energy cost by 26%) compared to providing exactly the same amount of electricity (30 kWh) and heat (45 kWh$_{heat}$) from the national electricity grid and natural gas boilers respectively. In the trigeneration scenario, if the heat is converted to chilled water (A) then there is an 8% reduction in CO_2e emissions (and a 4% energy cost saving) compared to using an electric chiller.

The CHP energy cost savings are based on a tariff of 10p/kWh for electricity and 3.5p/kWh for natural gas. The savings are very sensitive to the spark gap, the difference in price between the CHP input fuel tariff and the electricity tariff. This is discussed later in the chapter.

Table 7.15 shows how the results in Figure 7.19 change if natural gas is replaced by the lowest carbon biofuel available (recycled cooking oil). This has an emission factor of 0.06 kgCO_2e/kWh (one-quarter that of natural gas) and a fuel cost of 7p/kWh (twice that of natural gas). All of the options see an increase in energy costs of between 50% (CHP) and 200% ('one-generation').

	A Trigeneration (cooling)	B Cogeneration (heating)	C 'One-generation'
Emissions from grid equivalent	22	28	14
CO_2e savings	16	22	8
% CO_2e saving	72%	79%	57%
Energy cost from grid equivalent	£3.63	£4.75	£2.33
Energy cost saving	-£3.37	-£2.25	-£4.68
% energy cost saving	-93%	-47%	-201%

Table 7.15 CO_2e and cost savings for 100kWh of recycled cooking oil in biofuel CHP in the UK for different uses of heat

When does CHP become viable in buildings?

According to the Carbon Trust, '4,500 hours of high and constant heat demand is needed a year to make gas CHP economical'.[33] To put this into perspective, there are 8,760 hours in a year. A space heating system in an office building operating for 4 months a year from 7 a.m. to 6 p.m. Monday to Friday runs for just 950 hours.

Buildings account for less than 7% of the total CHP generating capacity in the UK,[34] because most buildings do not have a consistent annual demand for heat to make CHP viable. The vast majority of CHP capacity is used in industrial, chemical or manufacturing processes, which have high year-round heating requirements. Hospitals, hotels and leisure centres are buildings which do have a relatively high demand for heating all year round (a high 'base heat load') and are also used 7 days per week. Over 50% of the CHP systems installed in buildings in the UK are consequently found in these three building types.

Buildings that most commonly have CHP systems installed have the following characteristics:

- annual hours of CHP operation >4,500 (they require heat regularly)
- heat to electricity consumption ratio >2 (they use a lot of heat)
- winter to summer heat consumption ratio <5 (they use heat in summer).

This does not mean that CHP cannot be used in other building types, but it might be harder to justify. For example, office buildings need very little (if any) space heating in summer and the demand for domestic hot water (showers, washbasins, teapoints) is small. A mini CHP unit could be installed to provide domestic hot water all year round but, consequently, its overall contribution to reducing CO_2e emissions in the building would also be small.

If the office had air conditioning, then installing an absorption chiller to make use of heat generated in the summer would allow a larger CHP system to be installed. But, as Figure 7.19 shows, the conversion of heat into chilled water is not as efficient as using the heat directly for heating. The CHP plant can be switched off when there is no demand for the heat; however, if it is sitting idle it will take longer to recover the initial capital investment – and while it is switched off there is no carbon reduction benefit.

Assessing the financial viability of a CHP or trigeneration system requires detailed analysis to take into consideration:

- hourly heat, cooling and electricity demand profiles
- hours of operation of the CHP plant
- CHP and equipment efficiencies (including at part loads)
- size of thermal storage tanks
- capital cost of CHP plant
- spark gap (the price difference between CHP fuel and grid electricity)
- peak, off-peak and export electricity tariffs
- government incentives
- maintenance costs
- expected life of plant.

The analysis of CHP is very sensitive to small changes in any of the assumptions, particularly the spark gap (refer to box on page 173), turning what might appear to be a viable system into a white elephant. Appendix I provides some charts which can be used to make a quick estimate of the best case CO_2e and energy cost savings for gas CHP in the UK, based on the annual heat to electricity energy consumption ratio of the building.

CHP in Building X and Hotel Y

Table 7.16 shows the output from a simplified calculation, using seasonal heating energy profiles, to estimate the maximum CO_2e and cost benefits of gas CHP (with an electrical efficiency of 30% and heat output of 45%) in Building X and Hotel Y. Further details, including assumptions made, are given in Appendix I.

	CHP size (kWe)	Building heat from CHP	CO_2e saving $(kgCO_2e /m^2)$	Energy cost saving $(£/m^2)$	Indicative payback (years)	Net present cost (15 years)	£/tCO_2e: 15 years @ 5%
Building X							
Gas CHP	10	5%	0.6	£0.1	13	£725	£8
Gas CHP	100	39%	3.2	£0.4	27	£64,875	£135
Gas trigeneration	250	77%	9.3	£1.4	31	£237,125	£170
Hotel Y							
Gas CHP	100	35%	11.9	£1.8	7	-£105,532	-£59
Gas CHP	250	71%	19.6	£1.6	19	£105,800	£36
Gas trigeneration	250	71%	24.0	£1.8	23	£178,225	£50

Table 7.16 Maximum CO_2e reduction and cost/benefit of gas CHP in Building X and Hotel Y

The only options with reasonable paybacks (<15 years) are those sized to provide the base heat load. In Building X, this is for a small CHP system (10 kWe) providing domestic hot water – but this only reduces the operating carbon by 0.6%. The base load CHP option in Hotel Y (100 kWe) has a payback of 7 years and delivers an 11% reduction in operating carbon. To deliver more substantial CO_2e savings will require providing systems larger than the base heat load. Determining the optimum size of a CHP system for carbon reduction and financial benefit requires detailed analysis of building energy demand profiles and life cycle costs, which is too complex to discuss here. It is likely that, following such analysis, the actual system sizes will be smaller and consequently the actual CO_2e savings will be less than those shown in Table 7.16.

THE IMPORTANCE OF THE SPARK GAP

The cost analysis for CHP is very sensitive to assumptions for energy tariffs. Table 7.17 shows what happens to the paybacks for the systems in Table 7.16 with different tariffs.

		Base case		Increase gap		Decrease gap	
		Gas	Elec	Gas	Elec	Gas	Elec
	Tariff	3.5p	10p	2.5p	10p	3.5p	9p
	Spark gap	6.5p		7.5p		5.5p	
Building X							
Gas CHP	10 kWe	13		7		17	
Gas CHP	100 kWe	27		9		57	
Gas trigeneration	250 kWe	31		12		62	
Hotel Y							
Gas CHP	100 kWe	7		3		9	
Gas CHP	250 kWe	19		5		55	
Gas trigeneration	250 kWe	23		7		52	

Table 7.17 The influence of spark gap on payback periods for gas CHP in Building X and Hotel Y

A difference of just 2p/kWh in the spark gap can make a significant difference to the viability of a CHP system which is sized to provide more than the base load heating demand. For example, a 100 kWe gas CHP in Building X (which rejects 30% heat) has a 9-year payback with a spark gap of 7.5p and a 57-year payback with a spark gap of 5.5p.

It is critical when considering CHP to have a serious look at the energy tariffs and do some risk analysis on what might happen to these over the lifetime of the plant. The business case for CHP should not be hypersensitive to energy tariffs. If it is, it's probably not viable. Of the options shown, only the base load CHP in Hotel Y (100 kWe) has a payback of under 10 years for the decreased spark gap.

Exporting electricity to the grid (which reduces the effective spark gap because the export tariff is less than the consumption tariff) makes the financial case for CHP worse. Not using the heat effectively has the same effect. It's a fine balancing act to get everything right!

Biofuel CHP

The use of biofuel as a replacement for fossil fuels in engines is not a new concept. The inventor of the diesel engine noted in 1912 that farmers could run them on vegetable oil.[35] Biofuel CHP is similar in principle to gas CHP, the main difference being the need to deliver and store the biofuel on site.

There are four key questions to ask when considering biofuel CHP:

1. What is the CO_2e emission factor of the biofuel?
2. Is the biofuel from a sustainable source?
3. Will there be a reliable supply of affordable biofuel to the building for the next 20 years?
4. What is the cost of biofuel?

Biofuel is a renewable energy but is not necessarily a low carbon fuel (refer to Figure 7.20).[36] In this chapter the biofuel CO_2e factors are assumed to be 0.12 kgCO_2e/kWh for standard biofuel (biodiesel) and 0.06 kgCO_2e/kWh for recycled cooking oil.

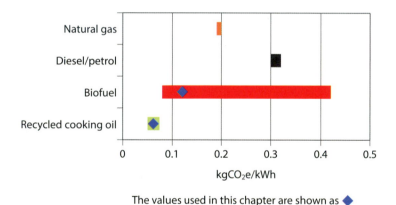

The values used in this chapter are shown as ◆

Fig 7.20 CO_2e emission factor range for biofuels compared to fossil fuels

While recycled cooking oil may have one-quarter of the CO_2e emissions of natural gas, there is clearly a limit to supply, particularly as the oil is also in demand from the transport sector. Many biofuels have CO_2e emissions greater than gas, and sometimes petrol and diesel as well. The type of crop and country of origin can have a significant impact on the potential CO_2e savings available from biofuel CHP.

There are also some significant environmental and social concerns regarding the impact of first generation biofuel crops on food prices and land clearing, and research is under way to make second and third generation biofuels commercially available.[37]

Biofuel CHP in Building X and Hotel Y

Table 7.18 summarises a simplified calculation to estimate the maximum CO_2e and cost benefits of biofuel CHP in Building X and Hotel Y. Further details, including assumptions made, are given in Appendix I.

	CHP size (kWe)	% of building heat from CHP	CO_2e saving ($kgCO_2e/m^2$)	Energy cost saving ($£/m^2$)	Indicative payback (years)	Net present cost (15 years)	$£/tCO_2e$: 15 years @ 5%
Building X							
Biofuel CHP	10	5%	1.3	-£0.2	Never	£49,050	£252
Biofuel CHP	100	39%	9.9	-£2.5	Never	£553,250	£373
Biofuel trigeneration	250	77%	26.0	-£6.0	Never	£1,451,775	£372
Hotel Y							
Biofuel CHP	100	35%	25.2	-£4.0	Never	£741,175	£196
Biofuel CHP	250	71%	52.9	-£13.0	Never	£2,228,850	£281
Biofuel trigeneration	250	71%	57.3	-£12.8	Never	£2,303,775	£268

Table 7.18 Maximum CO_2e reduction and cost/benefit of biofuel CHP in Building X and Hotel Y

The highest potential CO_2e reduction in Building X is 25% using biofuel trigeneration; however, the financial business case is not compelling, with an energy cost increase of 34%. In Hotel Y, a 55% CO_2e saving could be achieved for an energy cost increase of 72%. Table 7.19 shows the potential CO_2e savings if recycled cooking oil is used instead of typical biofuel.

Recycled cooking oil	CO_2e saving ($kgCO_2e/m^2$)
Building X	
CHP (10 kWe)	1.8
CHP (100 kWe)	14.9
Trigeneration (250 kWe)	38.5
Hotel Y	
CHP (100 kWe)	35.2
CHP (250 kWe)	77.9
Trigeneration (250 kWe)	82.3

Table 7.19 Maximum potential CO_2e reduction using recycled cooking oil CHP in Building X and Hotel Y

A large corporate office building in central London, with a GIA of around 60,000 m^2, can help put the theoretical maximum savings in Table 7.19 into perspective. The building has a 770 kWe biofuel trigeneration system which is equivalent to 128 kWe per 10,000 m^2 (Building X's system, at 250 kWe, is probably significantly oversized). In its first year of operation in 2011/12, using 310,000 litres of recycled cooking oil, it saved 550 tCO$_2$ (approximately 9 kgCO$_2$/m^2).[38] While this is expected to improve in future years it does suggest that the maximum potential carbon savings shown in Tables 7.18 and 7.19 are highly optimistic and unlikely to be realised in practice.

SHOULD BIOFUEL BE USED IN BUILDINGS OR TRANSPORT?

Biofuels are a finite resource – there is a limited amount of land available for their production. Second generation biofuels, such as recycled cooking oil, have an even more limited supply. Should this resource be used in buildings, which can obtain low carbon energy from a variety of sources including solar, wind, nuclear and biomass, or in transport, which has limited fuel options? We are unlikely to see wood pellet powered planes or cars.

The emission factor for diesel is 0.32 kgCO$_2$e/kWh (refer Table 1.1). 100 kWh of diesel (about 10 litres) used in a car, truck or train has emissions of 32 kgCO$_2$e. The consumption of 100kWh of recycled cooking oil (with an emission factor of 0.06 kgCO$_2$e/kWh) releases 6 kgCO$_2$e. If 100kWh of recycled cooking oil was used (in a blended mix) to replace 100kWh of diesel then the carbon saving would be 26 kgCO$_2$e. From Table 7.15 the best possible carbon reduction using 100 kWh of the oil in biofule CHP (Option B – no heat wasted) is 22 kgCO$_2$e.

The cost of commercial (red) diesel in January 2013 was around 0.7p/kWh (70p/litre) which is similar to the cost of biofuel. The cost increase of using 100kWh of biofuel in a vehicle is effectively zero compared to an increase of £2.25 (23p/litre) for biofuel in a CHP system. The cost to convert a vehicle to use a blend of biofuel and diesel is also negligible compared to the significant capital cost of installing a biofuel CHP system in a building.

Transport accounts for 20 to 25% of the UK's CO$_2$ emissions. It is clear that from a carbon and cost perspective all available biofuel should be used in transportation. Using biofuel in CHP systems is really an exercise in vanity (there is no compelling financial business case) and diverts a limited resource away from where it can be used more effectively and efficiently to reduce national CO$_2$ emissions.

7.9 WHAT IS THE MAXIMUM CONTRIBUTION OF ON-SITE SYSTEMS?

So far, each system has been considered individually. It is not possible to install all of these systems in the same building and add up the maximum savings because they either occupy the same space (e.g. PV and solar thermal panels) or they are meeting the same demand for heat (e.g. biomass boilers and gas CHP). Two scenarios are considered to estimate the maximum CO_2e savings that a combination of on-site renewable/low carbon energy systems could potentially make to Building X and Hotel Y:

1   maximum CO_2e saving
2   maximum CO_2e saving without fuel deliveries to site.

Table 7.20 (overleaf) shows the CO_2e reduction for each system individually and the combination of systems to estimate the two maximum CO_2e saving options.

The maximum possible CO_2e reduction due to on-site renewable systems in these buildings is 30% in Building X and 60% in Hotel Y. The bulk of this theoretical reduction would be due to the use of biofuel trigeneration. Hotel Y could also potentially achieve a 33% reduction using a combination of biomass boilers and PV.

If the use of biofuel or biomass is not possible, due to various constraints including access for delivery, noise from delivery trucks, storage constraints or air quality emission standards, then the maximum possible savings reduce to 14% in Building X and 28% in Hotel Y. It is important to note that these estimated savings are based on installing the largest possible renewable energy systems in the buildings. The systems are likely to be smaller in practice (and the CO_2e savings consequently lower) when capital costs, energy demand, export tariffs, maintenance costs, integration with HVAC systems and available floor/roof space are considered in more detail.

On-site renewables are not the silver bullet to significantly reduce the carbon footprint of buildings. They can play a part, but reducing the energy consumption of buildings first is fundamental. Investment in decarbonising the electricity grid through large-scale off-site renewables will clearly be necessary to practically deliver a 'zero carbon' building (refer to Figure 7.21).

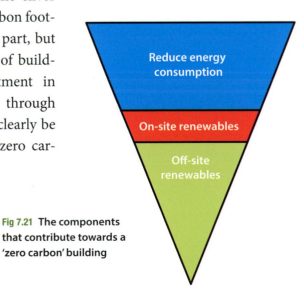

Fig 7.21 The components that contribute towards a 'zero carbon' building

	Heat	Electricity	Carbon footprint saving kgCO$_2$e/m^2	Reduction in building CO$_2$e	Option 1 Maximum CO$_2$ saving	Option 2 No fuel delivery
Building X						
Solar thermal	■		0.6	1%		
Biomass boiler	■		8.9	9%		
Heat pumps*	■		4.1	4%		
Photovoltaics		■	4.5	4%	Y	Y
Wind turbine		■	1.0	1%	Y	Y
Gas CHP	■	■	0.6	1%		
Gas trigeneration	■	■	9.3	9%		Y
Biofuel CHP	■	■	1.3	1%		
Biofuel trigeneration	■	■	26.0	25%	Y	
Option 1: Maximum CO$_2$ saving			**31.5**	**30%**		
Option 2: No fuel delivery			**14.8**	**14%**		
Hotel Y						
Solar thermal	■		1.9	2%	Y	
Biomass boiler	■		29.6	28%	Y	
Heat pumps**	■		7.5	7%		
Photovoltaics		■	4.5	4%	Y	Y
Wind turbine		■	1.0	1%	Y	Y
Gas CHP	■	■	11.9	11%		
Gas trigeneration	■	■	24.0	23%		Y
Biofuel CHP	■	■	25.2	24%		
Biofuel trigeneration	■	■	57.3	55%		
Option 1: Maximum CO$_2$ saving			**62.8**	**60%**		
Option 2: No fuel delivery			**29.5**	**28%**		

 * Based on CoP of 3.8 for combined ground and air source.

** Based on CoP of 3.6 for combined ground and air source.

Table 7.20 Summary of maximum CO$_2$e reduction due to renewable systems in Building X and Hotel Y

7.10 THE COST OF SAVING CARBON

Figure 7.22 shows the cost of carbon for the different systems evaluated in Building X and Hotel Y. This is based on a net present cost of the system divided by the CO_2e savings over a 15-year period. The variation for the heating systems is because Hotel Y has more demand for heat year round and, consequently, the capital cost per tCO_2e is lower. Appendix I provides charts for different evaluation periods and discount rates.

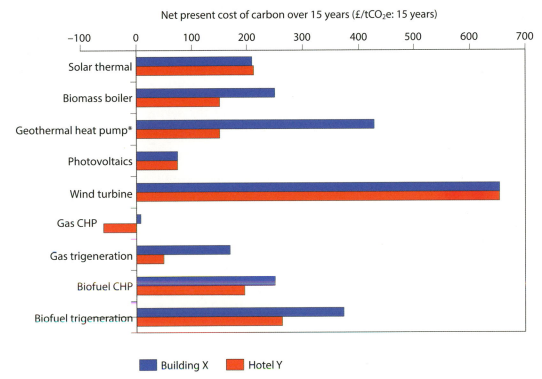

Fig 7.22 The net present cost per tCO_2e saved over 15 years for renewable systems in Building X and Hotel Y

The European Union Emissions Trading Scheme (EU ETS) puts the cost of carbon at somewhere between £10 and £20 per tonne.[39] The only system with a carbon cost less than £20 per tonne is gas CHP in Hotel Y – and that is not a renewable. If a carbon tax of around £15 per tonne was introduced (equivalent to 0.9p per kWh of electricity – a 10% increase on commercial UK tariffs in 2013) it would not significantly alter the financial viability of renewable energy systems in buildings.

To encourage building owners to install renewable energy systems, various governments have introduced incentives such as feed-in tariffs for electricity generated by photovoltaics and wind turbines. In 2011, the UK Government also introduced the world's first equivalent tariff for heating, called the Renewable Heat Incentive (RHI). Gas CHP and air source heat pumps were excluded on the basis that they are not renewable and biofuel CHP was excluded due to concerns about the sustainability of producing biofuel and using it in buildings instead of for transport.[40]

Applying the UK tariffs valid in January 2013 to Building X and Hotel Y has a major impact on the payback and net present cost of the systems, reducing some by over 60%. The tariffs typically cost between £100 and £400 per tonne of CO_2e saved depending on the type and size of system.

7.11 CONCLUSION

The purpose of this chapter was to put into perspective the maximum contribution that renewable and low carbon energy systems can make to reducing CO_2e emissions in typical non-domestic buildings. Some of the savings are disappointingly small – but it is important to have a realistic understanding of costs and benefits so that money can be invested in solutions that deliver the maximum CO_2e savings. The simple payback periods for most renewable energy options, ignoring any government incentives such as feed-in tariffs, are typically greater than 20 years, and some options never pay back the initial investment.

Reducing energy consumption in buildings (refer to Chapter 6) is therefore still the most important strategy for building owners, occupiers, designers and developers. This can be achieved at no additional cost (by changing controls and/or behaviours) or through investments with payback periods of less than 5 years, such as lighting upgrades.

On-site renewables should be selected based on the technical and commercial viability of a particular site – and not according to some arbitrary planning requirement. Government incentives are usually required to make many renewable systems commercially viable compared to fossil fuel alternatives. The latter are often heavily subsidised by governments and also have the benefit of almost a century of market development.[41]

Making it easy for building owners and developers to invest in off-site systems, and have the renewable energy attributed directly to them (and ensuring that the renewable energy benefit is not sold twice), would encourage investment in more cost effective renewable solutions.

Finally, a green building is not an energy guzzler with a few visible solar panels, wind turbines or biofuel deliveries. Adding renewable energy systems should be the icing on the cake of an efficient building, and not lipstick on a gorilla.

DECARBONISING THE GRID

Decarbonising the national electricity grid will be an essential component in achieving substantial reductions in the CO_2e emissions associated with buildings by 2050.

The approaches taken will vary in different countries but are likely to involve a mix of large-scale renewables (wind, solar, geothermal, hydro and biomass), nuclear power, gas turbines and carbon capture from coal power stations (if the technology proves to be technically and financially viable). Some factors to consider:

- Put wind turbines where it is windy and put solar panels where it is sunny.
- Where are we going to get all the biomass from?
- Nuclear is low carbon – but what about the risks, and how much will it cost to get rid of the waste safely over the next few thousand years and who will bear this cost burden?
- New extraction techniques are unlocking large shale oil and gas reserves which could not previously be extracted commercially – but there are concerns about potential groundwater contamination, seismic activity and methane leakage.
- There is still a lot of coal available so using it efficiently and capturing the carbon is going to be really important. If it is a choice between using coal or the lights going out, there is only one option that will prevail politically.

To get a better idea of the scale of this challenge in the UK read David MacKay's book *Sustainable Energy – Without the Hot Air*.[42] What is clear is that the UK can't live on home-grown renewables alone, even if energy consumption in buildings is reduced significantly.

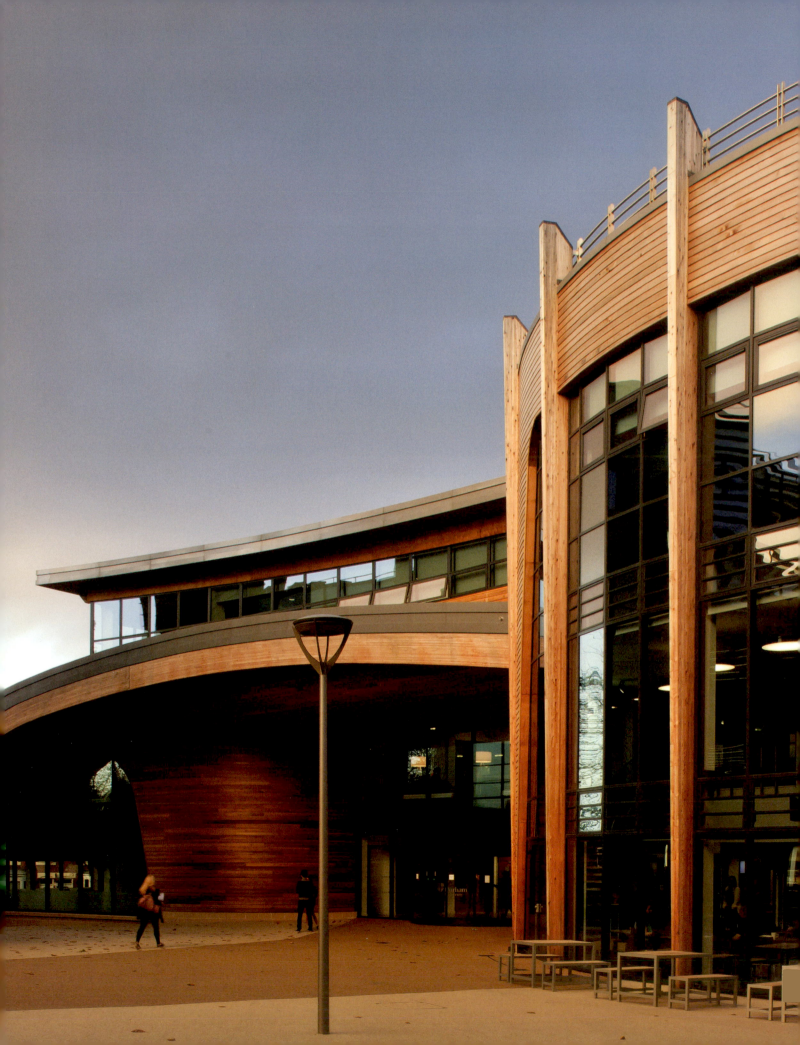

Chapter 8

Lower carbon materials

Look closely at the present you are constructing: it should look like the future you are dreaming.

Alice Walker, American author

In Chapter 3 the contribution of embodied carbon (ECO_2) to the whole life carbon footprint was discussed and typical values given for construction, fit-out and refurbishment of office buildings. This chapter looks at methods of reducing the embodied carbon by focusing on the components and materials that have the biggest impact. At the top of the list is concrete, which typically accounts for between 30 and 50% of the initial construction embodied carbon; however, fit-out components, which may at first glance appear minor, can also have a significant impact over the life of the building if they are replaced regularly.

8.1 ECO_2 BREAKDOWN AND KEY MATERIALS

Figure 8.1 (overleaf) shows an embodied carbon breakdown for a new 21-storey steel framed office building with three basement levels over a 60-year period. It assumes that the façade and central building services are replaced after 30 years and that a fit-out takes place every 15 years (including carpets, ceilings, partitioning and tenant services). The purpose is to illustrate the principle that embodied carbon must be considered over the lifetime of the building and not just during the initial construction. The lifespan of components should not be ignored.

This chapter provides guidance on reducing the embodied carbon of the following products and activities, which typically account for over 70% of the embodied carbon in the life cycle of office buildings:

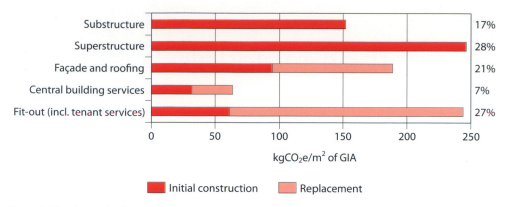

Fig 8.1 Indicative embodied carbon over 60 years for a 21-storey steel framed office building with three basement levels

- concrete
- steel
- timber
- masonry
- windows and curtain walling
- carpets
- plasterboard
- furniture
- external paving
- construction process and waste.

Building services (landlord and tenant) use combinations of metals and plastics and may account for between 5 and 10% of the whole life embodied carbon but, unfortunately, there is limited data available to provide meaningful guidance in this chapter. The wider uptake of environmental product declarations and/or further research should improve knowledge on the contribution of building services in a building's embodied carbon footprint, and how to reduce it.

All ECO_2 factors ($kgCO_2e/kg$) stated in this chapter for different materials are taken from the University of Bath's *Embodied Carbon: The Inventory of Carbon and Energy*, version 2 (ICE v2) unless noted otherwise. The stated range of uncertainty with the data, based on the embodied energy, is typically +/-30%.

While ICE v2 is widely used, and freely available, its use in this book is not intended to imply that it is more accurate than other databases. Alternative ECO_2 databases may give different results to those shown in this chapter. The measurement of embodied carbon is still in its early days and all databases have their limitations. The purpose of this chapter is to illustrate the principle of comparing the embodied carbon of different options and not to categorically state that one material is better than another, as to draw such conclusions depends on the quality and reliability of

OTHER ENVIRONMENTAL ISSUES WITH MATERIALS

There are clearly many other environmental issues to consider with materials other than carbon, but these are beyond the scope of this book. From a sustainability perspective, the ideal material or product has the following attributes:

- zero carbon emissions in its manufacture
- made from 100% renewable sources (unless the resources are abundant)
- non-toxic and non-polluting
- manufactured locally and transported via efficient vehicles
- appropriately durable and long lasting
- fully recyclable and/or reusable at the end of life
- ethically sourced
- zero ozone depletion and low global warming potential
- minimal use of water in water-stressed regions.

The assessment of these issues may be covered in Environmental Product Declarations and/or Ecolabelling schemes.[1]

the ECO_2 data used, how it is applied, and the boundary conditions assumed – refer Figure 3.6 in Chapter 3.

Currently ECO_2 factors tend to be only available for generic materials, and data on individual products is limited and often inconsistent. This means it is difficult to compare one supplier's product data against another's with confidence. The increased use of third party certified Environmental Product Declarations will be essential to improve the robustness of the embodied carbon assessment of buildings and materials.

8.2 WHAT IS THE LOWEST CARBON STRUCTURE?

The structure is the biggest component of the initial embodied carbon of a new building. Consequently, the various trade organisations representing concrete, steel and timber, all actively advocate the low carbon benefits of their products:[2]

- The steel industry promotes that steel buildings have lower embodied carbon compared to concrete and may also be lower than timber.
- The concrete industry states that the differences between concrete and steel buildings are quite small and insignificant when compared to operating CO_2 and that concrete can reduce operating carbon if its thermal mass properties are utilised.

- Proponents of timber claim that it is by far the lowest carbon material and can be considered to be carbon negative.

Can they all be right? Well, it all depends on what assumptions have been made in the calculations – particularly in terms of the emission factors, how efficiently the material is used and what happens at the end of life. Appendix J provides a summary of various case studies and analysis comparing the embodied carbon of steel and concrete framed buildings. This shows that there is currently no compelling evidence to prove that an efficient, economic design in steel is significantly better than an efficient, economic design in concrete.

The choice of structural form for a particular building is based on a variety of factors, including number of storeys, regularity of floor plates, clear span between columns, site accessibility, ground conditions, availability/capacity of local suppliers, programme, flexibility, adaptability, thermal mass, aesthetics, the experience and preference of the designers and contractors and, of course, capital cost. Embodied carbon is rarely a consideration in the selection of structural systems, particularly as the data sources and methodologies are so open to interpretation.

To avoid getting drawn into circular arguments about which material is best, a pragmatic approach is to choose the most efficient and economic structural solution and then focus on how to reduce its embodied carbon (and other environmental impacts) by:

- avoiding overdesign and waste to reduce the amount of materials used
- considering durability and flexibility for future uses to give the building a longer lease of life
- designing for easy demolition and reuse/recycling of components at the end of life
- specifying lower carbon versions of materials where possible.

REFURBISH OR REPLACE?

The considerations which influence the decision on whether to refurbish or replace an existing building include fitness for purpose, condition and expected life of the structure, heritage requirements and life cycle costs. Whole life carbon (operating and embodied) is also likely to become a factor in the future.

In Chapter 3, the comparison of embodied and operating life cycle carbon included a scenario of demolishing a building after 30 years and replacing it with a newer version. This showed that the impact on the whole life carbon footprint depends very much on whether the new building provides a significant improvement in operating energy efficiency. Flipping this around, if an existing building can be refurbished to significantly reduce operating carbon, then it is likely to be the lowest carbon solution.[3]

8.3 CONCRETE

Concrete is the world's most commonly used construction material[4] and is probably used in some form in every new office building. Steel framed buildings have concrete floor slabs and usually concrete core walls, and even a timber framed building will typically use concrete in the foundations. The main ingredients in concrete are cement, aggregate, sand, water and admixtures. The strength and properties of concrete are governed by the proportions of these in the mix – the higher the cement content the stronger and more durable the concrete.

The most commonly used cement is Portland cement, which accounts for around 95% of the embodied carbon of a typical C28/35 grade structural concrete mix. The simplest way to reduce the embodied carbon of concrete is to reduce the amount of Portland cement required in a mix by:

- avoiding over specification of strength
- using cement replacements
- use of admixtures.

CONCRETE STRENGTH

Concrete strength is usually specified based on the minimum compressive strength of a test cylinder or cube after 28 days. Cylinder strength is widely used in Europe except in the UK where cube strength is adopted. Consequently, in the UK both strengths are typically specified, with cylinder strength first. For example, a C32/40 concrete mix has a cylinder strength of 32 N/mm² and a cube strength of 40 N/mm².

Avoid over-specification

The grade (strength) of concrete required depends on where it is being used. Columns with high compressive loads require higher strength (and therefore higher cement content) than pad footings and ground floor slabs. Strength is not the sole determining factor for the concrete grade as the cement content also influences surface hardness durability and the minimum cover required to reinforcement. However, it is not uncommon for the strength of concrete to be over-specified in structural elements in office buildings.

The structural integrity of a suspended floor slab is primarily governed by the slab thickness (depth) and the steel reinforcement provided. For example, a C32/40 concrete mix increases the load capacity (kN/m²) of a 7.5 m two-way spanning 280 mm deep flat slab by less than 1% compared to a C28/35 concrete mix, but the embodied carbon is 10% higher.

Figure 8.2 shows the difference in embodied carbon for two different approaches to concrete specification in Building X, a hypothetical ten-storey concrete framed building.[5] A net saving of 6% was achieved by reducing the strength of the upper floors and ground slab by one grade. These two components account for over 70% of the total volume of concrete. Figure 8.2 also includes the embodied carbon due to reinforcement and formwork.

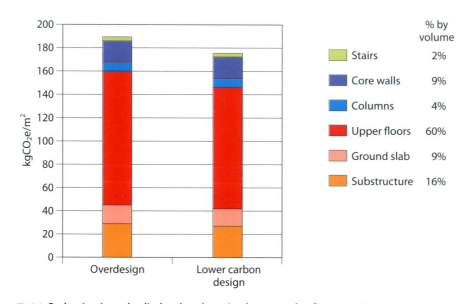

Fig 8.2 Reduction in embodied carbon by using lower grade of concrete in upper floors, slabs and footings in Building X

Concrete gains strength over time. On many building projects the programme does not allow work to stop for long periods while the concrete attains sufficient final strength (at 28 days), and achieving a minimum strength after a shorter period is often specified. This depends on the element and method of construction:

- Precast concrete: a minimum strength after as little as 8 hours is required to allow the precast element to be removed so that the next one can be poured in the same mould or casting bed as soon as possible.
- Floor slabs: in high-rise buildings the cycle for pouring a floor slab may be less than a week. To achieve the overall construction programme the temporary props usually need to be removed as soon as possible to allow the following trades (building services, etc.) to start work, and so a minimum strength after 7 days is required.

In both of these examples the cement content may be increased to ensure that the minimum short-term strength requirements are achieved. Careful consideration of the construction programme can reduce the need to over-specify short-term concrete strengths.

Increasing the cement content in exposed elements (e.g. façades, exposed slabs and foundations) to increase the durability is also fairly common, although the use of admixtures can help to increase surface hardness and reduce porosity without increasing cement content.

Cement replacement

The production of Portland cement is energy intensive and therefore expensive. Fortunately, a proportion of Portland cement can be replaced in concrete mixes with waste by-products from other industries, reducing both the embodied carbon and cost. The most commonly used are pulverised fly ash (PFA) and ground granulated blastfurnace slag (GGBS), although other materials are under development.[6] Cement replacement is widely used in standard concrete mixes because it is cheaper – the reduced embodied carbon is a free bonus.

The addition of cement replacement can alter the properties of concrete in a number of ways compared to a mix with 100% Portland cement (PC) including:

- colour
- lower early strength gain (parity is usually reached after 56 days)
- extended curing times
- lower heat gain during hydration
- reduced permeability
- increased sulphate resistance.

The lower early strength gain if high proportions of cement replacement are proposed is a key challenge for use in reinforced concrete as this can impact on the programme, and therefore on the project cost. Methods to address low early strength gain include the use of accelerating admixtures, insulated formwork and accelerated application of curing. Table 8.1 (overleaf) shows the typical and maximum practical proportions of GGBS and PFA used in standard concrete mixes in the UK.

Higher proportions can be used in specialised applications, such as deep sections where the heat of hydration (the heat given off as the concrete hardens) needs to be limited to prevent thermal cracking, or in marine applications where reduced permeability and sulphate resistance increases durability. The longer setting time

	GGBS	PFA
Waste by-product from	Steel manufacture	Coal power station
% of ready-mix concrete in the UK using product[7]	50%	20%
Colour	White/light grey	Dark grey
Typical proportion in concrete mixes	30%	15%
ECO_2 reduction in C32/40 concrete mix	18%	7%
Maximum practical proportion in concrete mixes	50%*	30%**
ECO_2 reduction in C32/40 concrete mix	39%	17%

* In fair faced concrete the limit is around 40% to prevent problems with discolouration and plastic cracking of the finished surface.[8]

** Up to 40% is acceptable in piling.

Table 8.1 Typical properties of cement replacement

of GGBS concrete can hinder surface finishing, which discourages its use in power floated floor slabs (e.g. warehouse floor slabs).

Figure 8.3 shows the reduction in embodied carbon using different proportions of cement replacement in all concrete elements in Building X. Table 8.2 shows typical cradle-to-gate ECO_2 factors for different concrete mixes.

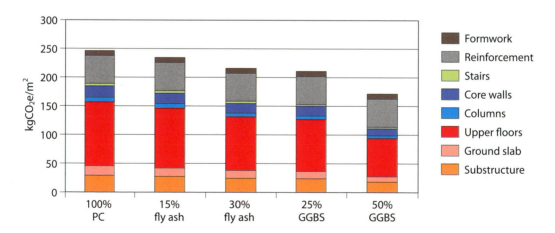

Fig 8.3 Reduction in structural embodied carbon using different proportions of GGBS and PFA in Building X

	ECO$_2$ factor (kgCO$_2$e/kg)					Comments
	100% PC	15% PFA	30% PFA	25% GGBS	50% GGBS	
GEN 0 (6/8 MPa)	0.076	0.069	0.061	0.06	0.045	Mass concrete/blinding
GEN 1 (8/10 MPa)	0.104	0.094	0.082	0.08	0.058	
GEN 2 (12/15 MPa)	0.114	0.105	0.093	0.088	0.065	
GEN 3 (16/20 MPa)	0.123	0.112	0.1	0.096	0.07	
RC 20/25	0.132	0.122	0.108	0.104	0.077	Reinforced concrete
RC 25/30	0.14	0.13	0.115	0.111	0.081	
RC 28/35	0.148	0.138	0.124	0.119	0.088	
RC 32/40	0.163	0.152	0.136	0.133	0.1	
RC 40/50	0.188	0.174	0.155	0.153	0.115	
PAV1	0.148	0.138	0.123	0.118	0.088	Outdoor paving
PAV2	0.163	0.152	0.137	0.133	0.1	Heavy duty outdoor paving

Table 8.2 Typical cradle-to-gate ECO$_2$ factors for concrete mixes in the UK (source: ICE v2)

Admixtures

Concrete usually contains small quantities (less than 1% by weight) of various chemicals (admixtures) to modify the properties of the mix in the fresh and/or hardened state. The most common are plasticisers to improve the flow of concrete when pouring (without having to add more water). Others include accelerating, retarding, air entraining and waterproofing admixtures.

The use of plasticisers enables a given strength of concrete and or water/cement ratio to be achieved with a lower cement content, reducing the embodied carbon by typically 5 to 10%.[9] Admixtures can also enhance the long-term durability of concrete.

Reinforcement, formwork and aggregates

Reinforcement typically accounts for 20 to 25% of the embodied carbon of a floor slab and around 40% of a column. Avoiding overdesign of the reinforcement will reduce embodied carbon, although leaving out reinforcement to reduce embodied carbon is not a good idea.

The formwork used to pour concrete accounts for up to 5% of the embodied carbon in a concrete structure. Maximising the number of times that the formwork is used, and then avoiding sending it to landfill are the two main methods of reducing the embodied carbon due to formwork.

Aggregate usually represents less than 5% of the embodied carbon in a structural concrete mix. The use of recycled aggregate, while reducing the consumption of natural resources (e.g. gravel beds, marine aggregates and crushed rock from quarries) has negligible impact on the embodied carbon.

Table 8.3 gives typical ECO_2 factors for these components of reinforced concrete.

	ECO_2 factor	Comment
Reinforcement	0.770 $kgCO_2e/kg$	Some data suggest that this could be less than 0.5 $kgCO_2e/kg$ in the UK[10]
18 mm plywood formwork	6 $kgCO_2e/m^2$	Epoxy finish and reused five times
Aggregate	0.005 $kgCO_2e/kg$	This could range from 0 to 0.05 depending on the source of aggregate[11]

Table 8.3 Typical cradle-to-gate ECO_2 factors for other components of reinforced concrete (source: ICE v2)

CEMENT PRODUCTION AND REABSORPTION OF CO_2

The production of cement (primarily Portland cement) is responsible for up to 5% of global greenhouse gas emissions.[12] About half of this is due to the combustion of fossil fuels and electricity in the various manufacturing processes and the remainder is due to the release of CO_2 when calcium carbonate (limestone) is calcinated and converted to lime (CaO), the primary component of cement ($CaCO_3$ + heat = CaO + CO_2).

When mixed in concrete, the cement will start to absorb CO_2 from the atmosphere in a process known as carbonation. This makes the concrete less alkaline. The high alkalinity of concrete is the primary mechanism to prevent the steel reinforcement from corroding. If the depth of carbonation reaches the reinforcement (typically 20 to 50 mm from the surface), then the rebar may start to corrode. As it does so it expands, causing chunks of concrete to break off (spall), exposing more rebar to air, which then rusts further. The integrity of the structure can then be compromised if repairs are not undertaken.

Approximately 20 to 30% of the CO_2 released in the calcination process is reabsorbed over a 60-year period in dense concrete, even after it has been crushed and reused elsewhere. This reabsorption is typically not included in the embodied carbon factors for concrete as it occurs over a long period and the rate of absorption will depend on how the concrete is used.

Magnesium oxide cements can provide a lower carbon alternative to Portland cement, particularly in low strength applications. Calcination occurs at a lower temperature (reducing the demand for heat energy) and when used in porous materials, such as pavers or blockwork, the CO_2 emitted during calcination is more quickly reabsorbed. Research and development continues in order to make them a commercially and technically proven alternative to Portland cement in structural applications.[13]

Conclusion

Structural engineers have a significant role to play in reducing the embodied carbon of concrete in buildings and need to consider the carbon implications of the decisions they make when designing and specifying these elements. Most options are either cost neutral or can lead to cost savings. Challenging the supply chain to provide Environmental Product Declarations for concrete, reinforcement and formwork will also assist in creating a market for lower carbon products.

8.4 STEEL

Steel is produced worldwide to standard grades and there is little that a structural engineer can do to reduce the embodied carbon of steel by specification. Steel contains both recycled steel and virgin steel with the proportions depending on the production methodology:[14]

- Primary steel (approximately 75% of global steel production) is produced by reducing iron ores to iron in a blast furnace and then converting to steel in a basic oxygen furnace. The main inputs are iron ore, coal, limestone and recycled steel.
- Secondary steel (approximately 25% of global steel production) is produced in an electric arc furnace from recycled steel.

There is considerable disagreement about which ECO_2 factors to use for steel, with published factors varying by more than 100%.[15] Much of this stems from the choice of boundary conditions and whether the benefit of the recycled content in the steel when installed or the benefit of the recyclability of the steel at the end of its life in the building, or both, or neither, is used. This will eventually be resolved. Table 8.4 shows typical cradle-to-gate ECO_2 factors for steel from the ICE database which can be used in the interim. Galvanising adds around 0.2 $kgCO_2e/kg$.

Type of steel	Typical recycled content	kgCO$_2$e/kg			
		General	Section	Bar/rod	Stainless
Typical UK/Europe	59%	1.46	1.53	1.40	
Typical rest of world	36%	2.03	2.12	1.95	6.15
Primary	13%	2.89	3.03	2.77	
Secondary	100%	0.47	0.47	0.45	

Table 8.4 Typical ECO$_2$ factors for steel (source: ICE v2)

Specification

Worldwide, about 83% of steel is recovered from waste because it is too valuable to throw away.[16] Specifying steel with a minimum recycled content on a building project therefore makes no real difference to global CO_2 emissions as it does not alter the steel industry's global recycling rates. This is different to specifying GGBS or PFA in concrete mixes, as these are waste products which would probably end up on slag heaps if they were not used by the concrete industry.

Higher strength steel has a greater strength to ECO_2 ratio than lower strength steel and should therefore be used whenever practical to reduce the weight of steel in a building. To motivate the supply chain, contractors and designers can specify that steelwork supplied to projects has an Environmental Product Declaration and request evidence of the measures being undertaken by the suppliers to reduce CO_2 emissions.

Reuse

Reusing steel from a demolished building will save embodied carbon provided it is used efficiently in the new building. The Building Research Establishment (BRE) estimates a 96% environmental impact reduction compared to using a new steel section.[17] Table 8.5 shows the proportion of recycling and reuse of steel from buildings in the UK.[18]

	Sections	Purlins and side rails	Cladding	Composite floor decking
Recycled	86%	89%	79%	79%
Reused	13%	10%	15%	6%
Waste	1%	1%	6%	15%

Table 8.5 End-of-life recycling and reuse rates for steel products (source: Tata Steel, 2012)

To encourage the reuse of steel elements in the future, new buildings should:

- use bolted rather than welded connections where practical to allow easier dismantling
- have steel members permanently marked with their strength grade.

Design efficiency – reducing the weight of steel used

It is unlikely that there will be a radical technological break-through that will dramatically reduce the amount of energy required to create steel (either from recycled steel or iron ore). Consequently, the most practical method of reducing the embodied carbon due to steel is to reduce the weight of steel used. The design utilisation ratio is a measure of how efficiently a structural element has been designed.[19] Structural designers and fabricators should be required to report the average utilisation ratio of steel framed buildings to demonstrate they are using materials efficiently (and consequently reducing embodied carbon). A benchmark of 75% could be adopted, although it is likely than some designs achieve values less than 50%. Further research is required to confirm an appropriate target and reporting mechanism.

8.5 TIMBER

Timber is a naturally occurring and renewable material that has been used in buildings for millennia. If sourced from certified sustainably managed forest plantations then it is almost carbon neutral, with some CO_2 emissions due to forestry activities, processing and transportation. The assertion that timber delivers carbon negative structures is based on storing (sequestering) carbon in the structure while replacement trees grow and absorb CO_2 from the atmosphere. However, what happens at the end of life of the timber element cannot be ignored – is it reused or recycled, used to generate energy in biomass power stations or sent to landfill (with or without methane capture to convert to biogas)? Appendix J provides indicative CO_2 emissions that can occur at the different stages in the life cycle.

Counting the carbon stored in timber as an alternative to making deeper reductions to the energy consumption or CO_2e emissions of a new building is an approach that does not have universal support. It is difficult to justify unless all of the assumptions regarding end of life in the future are realistically achievable, clearly stated and all of the life cycle CO_2e emissions are included in the embodied carbon calculation.

In 2011 around 30% of wood waste in the UK was sent to landfill, 27% used as biomass fuel and 28% used to create particleboard.[20] The landfill rates may reduce in the future, although this depends on how the timber is used in a building. Timber is incorporated into a range of engineered products, such as plywood, glulam beams and cross-laminated panels, and composite wood products, such as particleboard and MDF. Their manufacture uses energy and various chemicals (resins and glues) and these can complicate recycling or incineration at the end of life. Wood waste containing chemicals is typically either used as biomass (in power stations with appropriate emission abatement controls) or sent to landfill.

Product	kgCO$_2$e/kg			Uncertainty*
	Fossil fuel	Biomass	Total	
General (mix of timber products in UK)	0.31	0.41	0.72	–
Sawn softwood	0.2	0.39	0.59	-90% to +75%
Sawn hardwood	0.24	0.63	0.87	-93% to +54%
Glue laminated timber	0.42	0.45	0.87	-33% to +16%
Plywood	0.45	0.65	1.1	+/- 33%
Orientated strand board (OSB)	0.45	0.54	0.99	not known
Particleboard	0.54	0.32	0.86	-72% to +3%
MDF (medium density fibreboard)	0.39	0.35 (?)	0.74	not known
Hardboard (high density fibreboard)	0.58	0.51	1.09	-7% to +119%

* Based on range of embodied energy (MJ/kg).

Table 8.6 Typical cradle-to-gate ECO$_2$ factors for timber products excluding carbon storage (source: ICE v2)

Table 8.6 shows two cradle-to-gate ECO$_2$ factors (excluding carbon storage) for different types of timber:

- fossil fuel – the cradle-to-gate fossil fuel energy used to harvest, manufacture and transport products
- biomass – the emissions from manufacturing/process offcuts which are used for fuelling sawmills and kilns.

The range of uncertainty in the data is very large due to:

- a lack of high-quality data on timber in the UK and EU
- variations in moisture content of trees
- variations in energy consumption to manufacture the same timber products
- variations in the fuel mix (particularly in drying kilns).

Reused timber has about 75% lower environmental impact compared to new timber.[21] New timber can provide a low embodied carbon solution in office buildings provided it is:

- sourced sustainably
- designed to maximise design life
- manufactured with non-toxic chemicals and coatings to simplify recycling
- not sent to landfill at the end of life.

8.6 MASONRY

The most commonly used masonry products in the UK are clay brick and concrete block, but there is a vast array of alternative products that can be used (refer to box below). Table 8.7 shows the cradle-to-gate ECO_2 factors for a 300 mm thick insulated masonry wall. The value per m² of wall includes 10 mm mortar with a mix of 1 part cement to 5 parts sand – refer to Appendix J for calculations. In comparison, a 200 mm thick precast concrete wall with 100 mm insulation has an embodied carbon of 110 $kgCO_2e/m^2$.

Product	$kgCO_2e/kg$	$kgCO_2e/m^2$ (per 100 mm thick)	Uncertainty range
Fired clay brick	0.24	37	-80% to +100%
Concrete block – 8 MPa	0.063	10	+/- 30%
Mineral wool insulation	1.28	3	+/- 40%
Total		**50**	

Table 8.7 Typical cradle-to-gate ECO_2 values for a 300 mm thick insulated masonry wall (source: ICE v2)

ALTERNATIVES TO BRICK/BLOCK

The following could be used instead of clay bricks and concrete blocks in many applications:

- calcium silicate bricks
- multi-cellular clay walling systems
- hemp blocks
- recycled wood and cement insulated blocks
- compressed earth blocks
- mudbrick – sundried earth blocks
- cob/adobe – compressed mix of earth and straw
- straw bales
- stone (including gabion baskets)
- prefabricated timber and straw bale modules with lime render
- cast in situ hemp-lime walling
- compressed strawboard panels.

To reduce the embodied carbon of masonry, consider using:

- bricks/blocks with low life-cycle carbon (supported by an Environmental Product Declaration)
- reclaimed bricks
- lime mortars instead of cement mortars to allow easier reuse of bricks in the future
- the lowest strength blockwork appropriate to the purpose (e.g. internal non-loadbearing partitioning or external loadbearing wall)
- bricks and blocks with voids (holes and/or aerated) to reduce the volume of material
- unfired clay bricks (less than 25% ECO_2 of fired clay bricks)
- blocks with cement replacement (GGBS or PFA)
- blocks made from magnesium oxide cement (which absorbs CO_2 – refer to box on page 192).

8.7 WINDOWS AND CURTAIN WALLING

Glass in windows and curtain walling systems represents between 70 and 90% of the structural opening by area, but the framing supporting the glazing can account for half of the embodied carbon. While it is not currently possible to specify a low carbon glass, asking for Environmental Product Declarations from suppliers may encourage further improvements in carbon reduction in the manufacturing process. Designers and contractors have much more influence on the embodied carbon when it comes to selecting the framing system.

Windows

Each 3 mm of glass has an embodied carbon of 6.8 $kgCO_2/m^2$. Table 8.8 shows the values for a typical double glazed window.[22] The frames in this example account for between 40 and 95% of the embodied carbon of the window unit. The expected life and maintenance requirements also need to be taken into account when deciding on a suitable frame.

	kgCO$_2$
Aluminium frame	279
PVC frame	110–126
Aluminium clad timber frame	48–75
Timber frame	25
Krypton filled add	26
Xenon filled add	229

Table 8.8 Typical cradle-to-gate ECO$_2$ values for a 1.2 m × 1.2 m double glazed window unit (source: ICE v2)

Curtain walling

A typical curtain wall framing system comprises glazing and extruded aluminium mullions and transoms. Aluminium has high embodied carbon (>9 kgCO$_2$e/kg). The structural component of the mullions and transoms can be replaced with steel or timber to reduce the embodied carbon of the façade system (refer to Figure 8.4). There are a variety of composite curtain walling systems available which utilise timber supports.

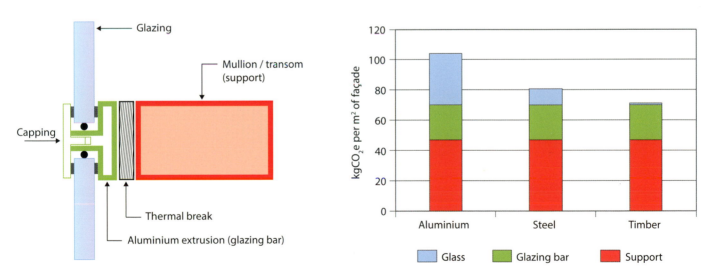

Fig 8.4 Typical ECO$_2$ breakdown for double glazed curtain walling system using different materials for the mullion and transom supports

8.8 CARPET

Floor finishes can have a significant impact on the embodied carbon footprint of an office building, particularly if they are replaced every 7 to 10 years. Currently, almost 600,000 tonnes of flooring is disposed of each year in the UK, of which less than 2% is recycled. A small quantity is incinerated, but over 90% goes to landfill.[23] Carpet accounts for 71% of this waste, laminate 13%, vinyl 6%, with the remainder distributed between ceramics, rubber, wood and linoleum.

Table 8.9 shows typical ECO_2 factors for different types of carpet. These should be treated with caution as there is a lack of reliable data available. It is likely that new carpets will have lower ECO_2 values.

Carpet type	Pile weight (g/m²)	Total weight (g/m²)	kgCO₂/m²	kgCO₂/kg
Nylon carpet (polyamide) (with tufted surface pile and woven fabric backing)	300	1,477	6.7	4.5
	500	1,837	9.7	5.3
	700	2,147	12.7	5.9
	900	2,427	15.6	6.4
	1,100	2,677	18.4	6.9
Nylon (polyamide) carpet tiles (with bitumen backing)	300	4,123	7.75	1.9
	500	4,373	10.7	2.4
	700	4,623	13.7	3.0
	900	4,873	16.7	3.4
	1,100	5,123	19.7	3.8
Polyethylterepthalate (PET)	–	–	–	5.6
Polypropylene	–	–	–	5.0
Polyurethane	–	–	–	3.8
Rubber	–	–	–	3.6 to 7.5
Wool	–	–	–	5.5*
Felt (hair and jute) underlay	–	–	–	1.0
Saturated felt underlay (with asphalt or tar)	–	–	–	1.7

* Other LCA software suggests this value could be over five times greater.

Table 8.9 Typical cradle-to-gate ECO_2 factors for carpet (source: ICE v2)

To reduce the embodied carbon of carpet:

- use heavy duty carpet in high wear areas to extend lifespan
- try not to get too carried away with garish colours – many perfectly functional carpets are thrown away because they have fallen out of fashion

- specify carpet with a lower yarn content (note: loop pile usually contains less yarn than cut pile)
- choose a carpet with a minimum of 25% recycled content from post-consumer waste. Carpet tiles with over 50% recycled content are available[24]
- avoid the use of strong carpet adhesives to allow carpet tiles in high wear areas to be replaced (or rotated with tiles from low wear areas)
- reduce offcuts waste – in the UK, typically 20% of carpet delivered to site is wasted, good practice can reduce this to 10%[25]
- use suppliers who have a product take-back scheme at the end of life to maximise recycling of carpets
- request suppliers to provide Environmental Product Declarations.

FROM CARPET TILES TO GLOBAL MODEL FOR SUSTAINABLE PRODUCTS

Interface manufactures carpet tiles for commercial buildings. In 1994, their CEO, Ray Anderson, realised that their products were made from unsustainable materials (oil by-products) and that millions of tonnes of old carpet were being sent to landfill each year. They were using the standard 'take–make–waste' manufacturing model. Ray decided to transform the company with a vision to eliminate its negative environmental impact.

Interface's model for improving the sustainability of the company and its products is summarised as: [26]

1 **Eliminate waste**: eliminate all forms of waste in every area of business.
2 **Benign emissions**: eliminate toxic substances from products, vehicles and facilities.
3 **Renewable energy**: operate facilities with 100% renewable energy.
4 **Close the loop**: redesign processes and products to close the technical loop using recovered and bio-based materials.
5 **Resource efficient transportation**: transport people and products efficiently to eliminate waste and emissions.
6 **Sensitise stakeholders**: create a culture that uses sustainability principles to improve the lives and livelihoods of all stakeholders – employees, partners, suppliers, customers, investors and communities.
7 **Redesign commerce**: create a new business model that demonstrates and supports the value of commerce based on sustainability.

Interface doesn't have all the answers yet, but by setting clear goals, and establishing the culture to deliver them, they are well on the way. Since starting down this path they have reduced costs and increased market share, demonstrating that embracing sustainability principles can go hand in hand with commercial success.

8.9 PLASTERBOARD

Plasterboard is manufactured from either mined gypsum or from synthetic gypsum, a by-product of the flue gas desulphurisation of coal-fired power station emissions. The recycled content of UK plasterboard products is typically around 76% and plasterboard is 100% recyclable.[27] Table 8.10 shows typical ECO_2 values for plasterboard.

	$kgCO_2/kg$	Thickness	Density	$kgCO_2/m^2$
Plasterboard	0.39	12.5 mm	650	3.2
Plaster	0.13	2 mm	1,120	0.3

Table 8.10 Typical cradle-to-gate ECO_2 of plasterboard (source: ICE v2)

To reduce the embodied carbon of plasterboard:

- consider demountable and reusable partitions instead of permanent plasterboard walls
- specify products with a minimum recycled content of 80%
- reduce waste (see below)
- request suppliers to provide Environmental Product Declarations
- use suppliers who have a plasterboard waste recovery programme
- avoid installing ceilings and instead expose the floor soffit (which can also have a thermal mass benefit).

Typically, 10% of plasterboard is wasted on site (thereby increasing the embodied carbon by 10% due to the extra material required).[28] This can be reduced to around 5% by:

- designing for standard board sizes
- minimising over-ordering
- accurate measurement and pre-cutting off site
- just-in-time delivery
- adequate dry storage
- reuse of offcuts.

8.10 FURNITURE

There is limited information, a lack of understanding and a fragmented approach to carbon footprinting in the furniture industry. A study in 2011 by the Furniture Industry Research Association[29] identified a number of concerns relating to the methodologies used, the number of products assessed, and the difficulty in getting accurate data from the global furniture supply chain.

Figure 8.5 summarises some of the embodied carbon assessments from the study. This determined that it was not possible at that time to establish embodied carbon benchmarks for different types of furniture. The study noted that:

In the absence of any carbon footprint benchmarks in the furniture industry for either individual products or for businesses, and with the danger of inconsistent representation of source data, it is impossible to make legitimate quantitative comparisons solely based on manufacturers' self declarations when evaluating tender submissions.

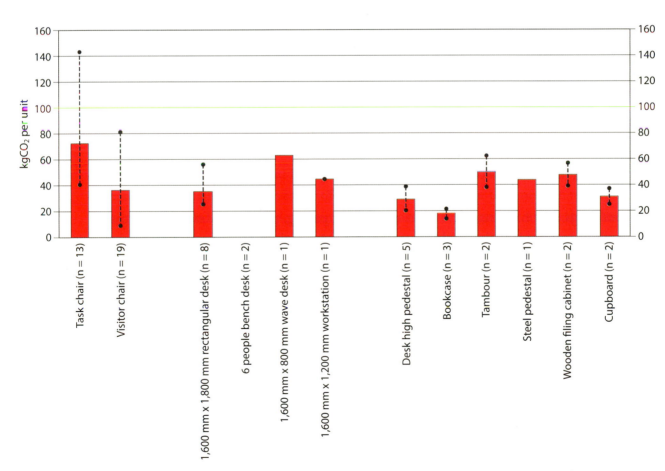

The black dotted lines denote the variation of data and 'n' stands for the number of products that the data are derived from.

Fig 8.5 **Summary of total average carbon footprints for office furniture (source: Furniture Industry Research Association)**

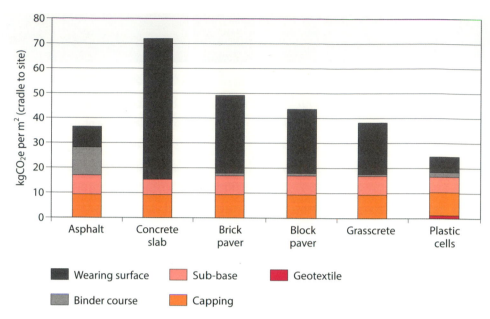

Fig 8.7 Typical cradle-to-site ECO$_2$ per m² for different pavement options

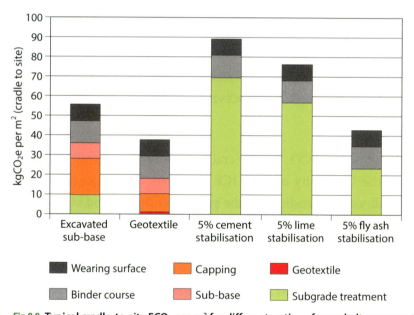

Fig 8.8 Typical cradle-to-site ECO$_2$ per m² for different options for asphalt pavement on weak subgrade

comparison of some potential treatment options for a standard asphalt pavement on a weak subgrade. Cement stabilisation of the subgrade has the highest embodied carbon but by using a fly ash mix instead (4% PFA + 1% lime) this can be halved.

In the UK, the introduction of landfill tax and the aggregate levy has led to the reuse of as much site material as possible (utilising methods including geotextiles and soil stabilisation). The environmental and financial benefit of reducing both the exporting of materials off site (generating waste) and the importing of materials (consuming natural resources) would also need to be considered, as well as the embodied carbon.

The methods of reducing the embodied carbon of external paving include:

- in permeable pavements, avoiding the use of bitumen or cement bound courses[31]
- using PFA or GGBS instead of cement in soil stabilisation, hydraulically bound materials and concrete mixes
- using vegetable-based emulsion in the surface dressing (laid when temperatures >10 °C)[32]
- using recycled products – brick pavers, asphalt pavers, etc.
- considering alternative materials to asphalt, such as C-Fix carbon concrete which utilises a thermoplastic heavy duty binder made from an oil refinery waste product.

8.12 CONSTRUCTION PROCESS AND WASTE

The construction process (site activities and transportation) can account for an additional 10 to 15% of the cradle-to-gate embodied carbon of the construction materials. Waste generated during construction can add a further 3 to 5% to the total. Any steps taken to reduce these will also save cost.

Construction process

The report *Carbon: Reducing the footprint of the construction process*[33] provides an estimated breakdown of CO_2 emissions in England due to construction processes and associated transport in 2008 (refer to Figure 8.9 overleaf). This is based on total emissions of 5 million tCO_2, which is equivalent to 47 tCO_2 per £million of contractors' output.

The same report proposed a series of actions that the UK construction industry could adopt to reduce CO_2 emissions associated with construction processes and transport by 15% including:

- energy efficient site accommodation
- efficient use of construction plant
- earlier connection to the electricity grid
- good practice energy management on site

- on-site measurement, monitoring and targeting
- fuel efficient freight driving and renewable transport fuels
- use of construction consolidation centres
- renewable (low carbon) biofuels
- reduction in transport of waste
- business travel fleet management
- good practice energy management of corporate offices.

Further details on these items are provided in Appendix J.

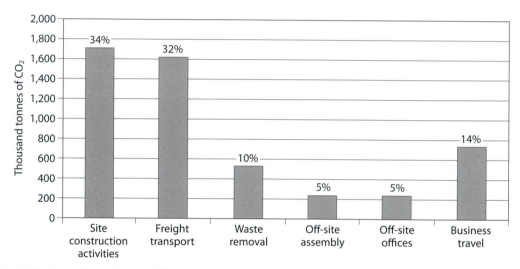

Fig 8.9 Estimated breakdown of CO_2 emissions from construction processes and associated transport in England in 2008 (source: Strategic Forum for Construction and the Carbon Trust, 2010)

Waste

Where there's muck there's brass.

Waste contributes to whole life embodied carbon through:

- manufacture and delivery of materials to site which are subsequently not used
- transportation of waste away from site
- energy to recycle into other products
- CO_2 and methane released if sent to landfill.

Reducing waste saves money and reduces natural resource consumption and CO_2 emissions. The car industry in the EU was forced by legislation to re-engineer its products to enable 85% recycling. This was greeted with significant grumbling and doom-mongering by the car makers and politicians in 1999. The car makers subsequently found lots of smart solutions to achieve the target and deliver cost savings at the same time.[34] The building industry is, on a voluntary basis, starting to rethink design and construction techniques to minimise waste and maximise the use of recycled or reclaimed products.

In the absence of legislative waste targets, a key step to reducing waste on a project is for the client to establish targets and to contractually commit the design and construction teams to achieving and reporting against these. After establishing the requirements, the teams can then get on with working out smart solutions to deliver them.

Table 8.12 shows the key steps to reducing waste during design and construction.

Key step	Actions
Waste targets	Establish a waste policy and targets at the start of the project. Refer to Appendix J for sample clause.
Design out waste	• Eliminate unnecessary elements. • Standardise sizes and details to reduce offcuts. • Reduce complexity to simplify construction process. • Evaluate the reuse and recycling opportunities of materials before specifying. • Maximise the reuse of demolished materials on site. • Consider off-site fabrication of buildings or elements to reduce waste.
Identify quick wins	Identifying quick wins is essential. By implementing good practice on three or four key waste streams on a project (typically those which occur in the largest quantities) it is possible to increase overall recycling rates by more than 20%, and make a cost saving.[35] Potential materials are concrete, metal, timber, packaging, ceramics, excavated soil, plasterboard, plastics, insulation and furniture.
Prepare and implement a Site Waste Management Plan	• Define responsibilities and actions to prevent, reduce and recover waste. • Identify waste arising, reuse and recycling routes. • Establish training requirements at every level of the waste supply chain. • Record waste movements and benchmark against best practice.
Logistics and materials procurement	• Set up a logistics plan and utilise just-in-time delivery. • Consider the use of Construction Consolidation Centres. • Reduce the amount of surplus materials by ordering the correct amount at the right time. • Provide safe, secure and weatherproof materials storage areas to prevent damage and theft. • Establish take-back schemes with suppliers to collect surplus materials. • Engage with the supply chain to supply products and materials using minimal packaging and segregate packaging for reuse.

Table 8.12 **Key steps to reducing waste during construction (source: adapted from WRAP)**

8.13 SUMMARY

Measuring and reducing the embodied carbon of buildings is still an emerging field and further research is required. Data is patchy, has a wide range of uncertainty (+/-30% is as good as it gets) and is usually only available for generic materials rather than products from specific suppliers. Until Environmental Product Declarations are widely available, produced using consistent methodologies, and independently verified, it will be difficult to compare the embodied carbon of one supplier's product with that of another. In the interim, common sense has to be applied instead.

The process of reducing embodied carbon can be summarised as follows:

- Design for low carbon by considering the type of materials, their efficient use and their expected life.
- Choose low carbon versions of the materials.
- Minimise wastage on site and design for deconstruction (reuse/recycling at end of life).

The specific steps to reduce embodied carbon will depend on the building design, the materials used and how they are assembled. In all cases there will be opportunities to make savings. Targeting the biggest components will deliver the majority of the benefits. On a typical office building project, by adding all these savings together, embodied carbon reductions of up to 20% should be achievable with little or no additional capital cost. These measures can be identified in the early design stages of projects using simple assessments (similar to developing a preliminary cost plan).

The primary material to focus on is concrete, which is found in all office buildings. It is probably the only material where the project team can directly control the ingredients used in the product and, by doing so, reduce an office building's initial embodied carbon by between 5 and 10%. The debate surrounding steel versus concrete structural frames is an unwelcome distraction; both types have similar overall embodied carbon footprints and both will continue to be used in buildings for economic and technical reasons.

WHY BOTHER?

The measurement and reduction of embodied carbon is not currently mandatory in most countries and is consequently rarely considered on most building projects. While it is possible that some form of embodied carbon legislation will be introduced for building construction in the future (or carbon taxes will increase some material costs), instead of waiting for the stick to arrive there is a carrot to be taken now. Embodied carbon can provide a useful proxy for the efficient use of resources – reducing embodied carbon reduces the resources and energy used in the construction and refurbishment of office buildings, which in turn reduces costs. By tackling embodied carbon now, designers and contractors can gain competitive advantage. That is probably reason enough to start.

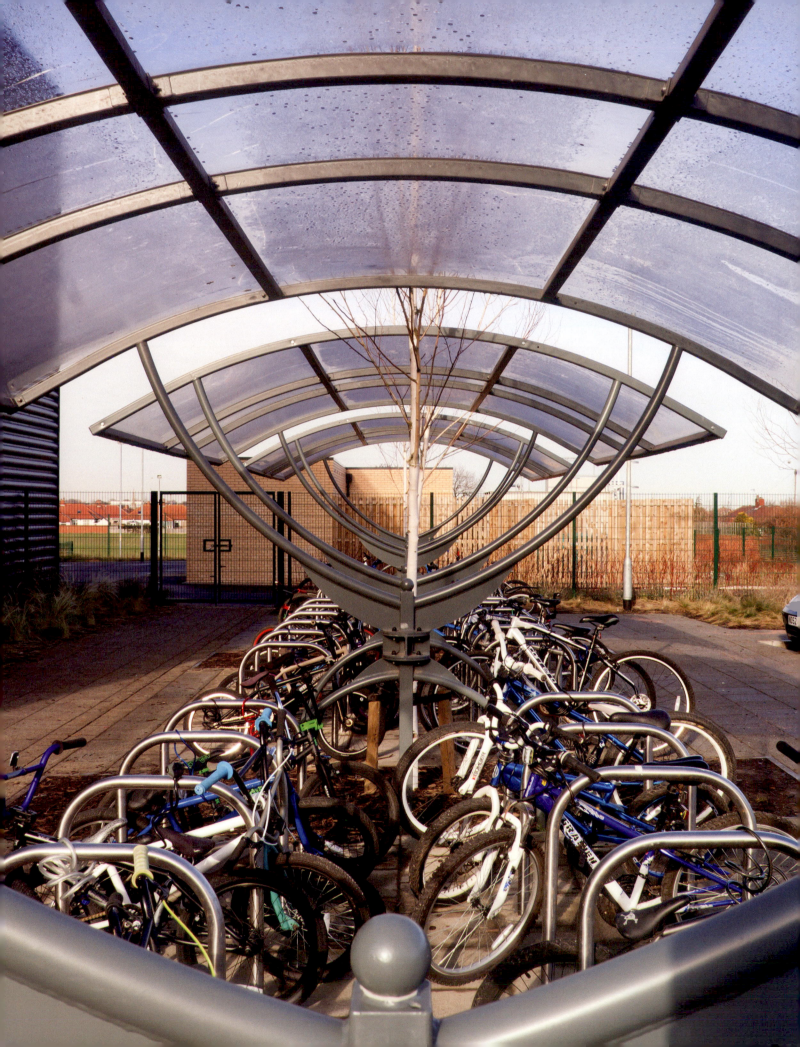

Chapter 9

Green travel

A journey of a thousand miles begins with a cash advance.
Bumper sticker

Chapter 4 showed that the CO_2e emissions due to people commuting between home and work can be greater than the CO_2 emissions due to the energy consumption of their office building. How people choose to get to work is primarily determined by the time, cost and convenience of their transport options. The location of a building, including its proximity to cheap car parking and a reliable public transport network, will have more influence than the number of cycle racks provided in the basement.

9.1 MODES OF TRAVEL

Figure 9.1 (overleaf) shows how people travelled to work in the UK in 2009.[1] Cars account for two-thirds of all commuting trips, and for 85% of these trips the car had only one occupant. The data is reasonably consistent across the UK, except in London where car use drops to 37% and public transport increases to 48%. For business trips, the use of cars increases to 78% in the UK.

A survey in 2002/03 found that 36% of those who usually travel to work by car or motorcycle would find it very or quite easy to get to work by other means, while 57% would find it difficult.[2] The most common reasons for the latter were:

- not believing that it was possible to do the journey by public transport (47%)
- the distance being too great (30%)
- poor public transport connections (29%)
- unreliable public transport (19%).

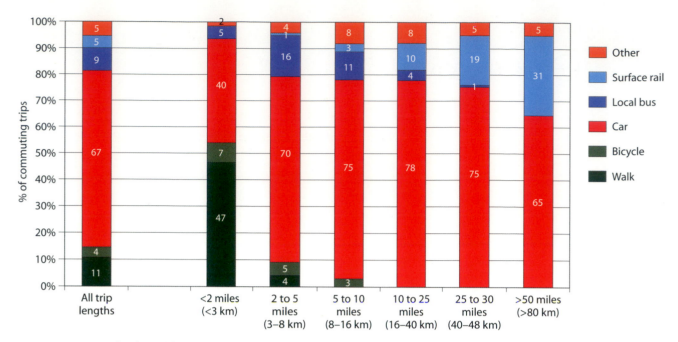

Fig 9.1 Mode of travel for commuting trips in the UK for different trip lengths (source: DfT, 2011)

While building owners, developers and designers have limited influence on the travel choices of the building occupants, there are numerous initiatives that can be implemented to reduce the carbon emissions associated with commuting, many of which can also be applied to business travel. These are often documented in a Travel Plan, which may be required as part of the planning approval process.

9.2 WALKING

The survey in Figure 9.1 shows that when the distance is under 2 miles (3 km) then around 50% of people walk to work. When the distance is 2 to 5 miles (3 to 8 km) this falls to under 2%. The following initiatives could encourage more walking:

- providing lockers and changing facilities
- relaxing the dress code
- ensuring safe pedestrian access to the building
- making occupants aware of urban walking route planners
  (e.g. www.walkit.com and www.livingstreets.org.uk)
- promoting a 'Walk to Work Week' with incentives for occupants who participate, for example, a free breakfast.

9.3 CYCLING

A distance of up to 10 miles (16 km) is a reasonable distance for people to cycle to work. All office buildings should make sensible provision for cyclists, matched to the likely current or future demand. This will depend on factors such as the building's location, topography (flat or hilly), climate, cycle paths, road safety and proximity to good public transport. Providing one cycle rack for every ten occupants might score points in rating tools but could be overkill in some locations and insufficient in others.

To encourage the uptake of cycling consider:

- cycling facilities (for all occupants who want them):
  - storage – secure, safe and accessible bike parking facilities
  - changing – good quality changing, showering and locker facilities
  - repair – provide or subsidise bike repairs near the building
- information:
  - produce a cycling route map for the building and make this available in hard copy and on a website. The safest, easiest and most pleasant cycle routes to the building may be different to the main routes motorists use, so draw on the knowledge of existing cyclists and local cycling organisations to prepare this
  - make occupants aware of web-based bike buddy schemes[3]
- incentives:
  - offset the cost of bikes and cycling equipment through cycle purchase schemes[4]
  - implement reward and incentive programmes to encourage cycling such as 'cycle to work' days[5]
  - provide free safe cycling courses for staff – don't assume that everyone is a confident cyclist, particularly in busy city centres.[6]

9.4 PUBLIC TRANSPORT

If the building is located near to reliable, clean, safe and economic public transport then people are likely to use it. The more routes and greater frequency of services, the higher the uptake will be. If suitable public transport is available close to the building then the following initiatives can be considered to increase its uptake:

- facilities:
  - create safe access to public transport services (e.g. lighting of pathways at night) and promote the use of these routes to occupants and visitors

- – in business parks, establish shuttle buses to connect to the nearest pub-
    lic transport hub
- incentives:
    - – introduce flexible hours to take advantage of the lower cost of off-peak
        fares
    - – provide interest-free loans for the purchase of season tickets
- information:
    - – provide real-time information on public transport timetables (and any
        service disruptions) on a display screen in reception
    - – prepare an information sheet with a map, showing public transport
        routes and typical frequency of services
    - – make occupants aware of public transport planning tools showing travel
        times, timetables and journey routes.[7]

9.5 CARS

If the building is in a city centre with lots of public transport, traffic congestion and
expensive car parking then most people will avoid using cars. If the building is in a
rural location with limited public transport then there may be no practical alternative
to driving to work. If a car is needed during the day for business travel then driving
to work may also be unavoidable.

Reducing the amount of car parking provided for an office building is an effective way of encouraging people not to drive to work and scores points in BREEAM,
LEED and Green Star rating tools. However, if there are not many viable alternatives
to driving (i.e. limited public transport) then this will also encourage people not to
work in that building. Clearly, a balance needs to be struck, recognising the role of the
car in society, while also aiming to minimise its impact.

To reduce the CO_2e emissions associated with the use of cars, the following initiatives could be considered:

- car parking on site:
    - – provide cheaper parking for car-sharing schemes and/or smaller, fuel
        efficient cars
    - – offer occupants an incentive to give up parking spaces/permits (and
        convert them to high-quality cycle facilities or green spaces)
    - – install subsidised electric car charging points
- company and private car use:
    - – provide fuel efficient company cars (including electric cars)

- set mileage allowances based on fuel efficient car costs (don't pay higher rates for larger engine sizes)
- make company cars available as pool cars during the day to reduce the need for staff to take a car to work
- maintain cars regularly and keep tyres at the correct pressure
- directors of companies have to join in. Driving to work in gas-guzzling status symbols and then lecturing others about environmental sustainability might be viewed by some as lacking in credibility

- staff incentives:
  - set up or join a car-sharing database for the whole building or groups of buildings (this does not have to be limited to individual companies)[8]
  - establish flexible working arrangements to avoid congestion during peak commuting hours (traffic jams increase fuel consumption)
  - offer free one-hour Smarter Driving lessons to all staff. Data from the Energy Saving Trust shows that this can lead to fuel savings up to 15%.

9.6 TELECOMMUTING

An alternative to commuting to an office is to work from home for some or all of the working week. This requires a combination of flexible and home working policies supported by appropriate information technology (including web conferencing). Various surveys have shown increased productivity and reduced sick leave due to utilising flexible working and telecommuting.[9] While it may not suit all businesses, working from home just one day a fortnight reduces commuting emissions by 10%.

9.7 SUMMARY

Commuting travel emissions have a significant impact on the carbon footprint of a building but are rarely given much importance in the low carbon design and operation of office buildings. Many of the initiatives to reduce transport carbon are relatively simple, and have other benefits including improving health and well-being (no one gets fit sitting in a car), reducing congestion and accidents, and saving money.

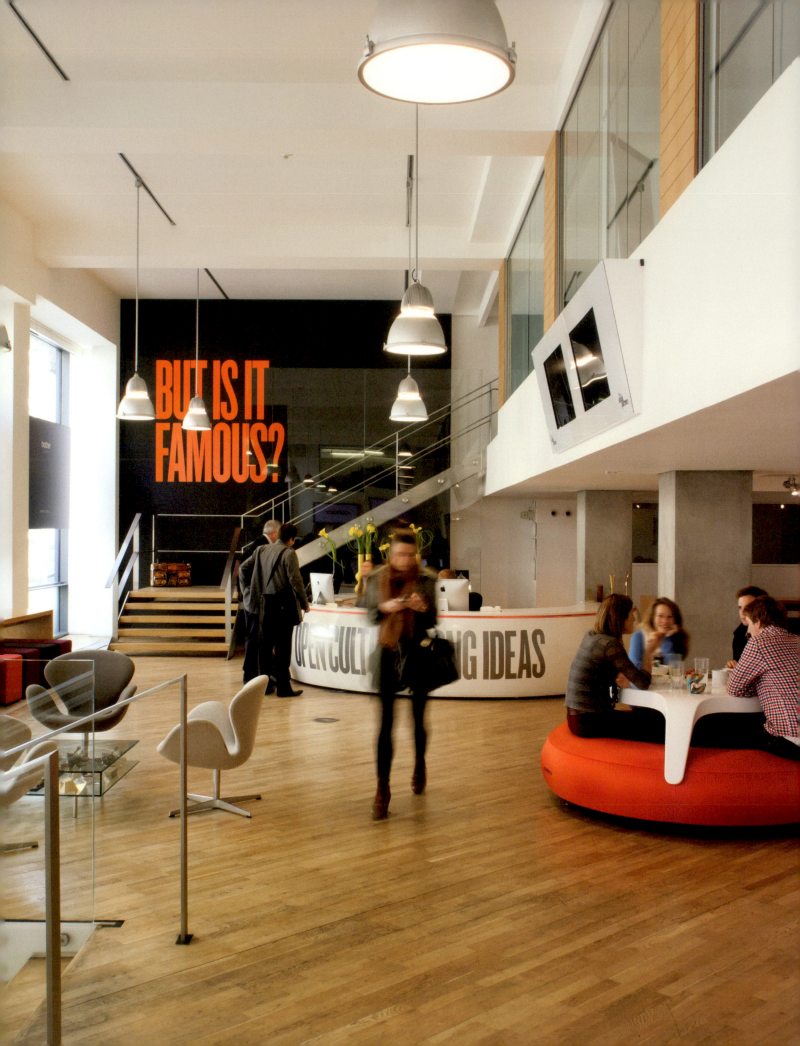

Chapter 10

Making the business case

We're not going to save the planet by putting our country out of business.

George Osborne, Chancellor of the Exchequer, UK

Conservative Party Conference, 2011

(John Maynard) Keynes's most important lesson is to let go of inherited ideas. If we cling to the panaceas of earlier times, we risk losing the civilisation we have inherited.

John Gray, political philosopher

BBC News Magazine, www.bbc.co.uk.news/magazine/, 22 July 2012

To radically improve energy efficiency and reduce its carbon footprint, the property industry needs to make changes which will require investment in both capital and people. In making a business case for such investment it is necessary to demonstrate to the decision makers in an organisation a compelling financial return, preferably with low risk and worthwhile additional benefits, such as enhanced corporate reputation.

In many organisations it may be difficult to recognise and account for revenue savings arising from capital expenditure in energy reduction. An additional challenge in commercial offices is the question of who gets the energy cost savings, landlord or tenant (which will depend on the leasing arrangements).

This chapter does not describe how to prepare a business case. Instead, the aim is to summarise some of the main drivers for, and barriers to, greener and lower carbon office buildings that might be incorporated into a business plan presented to decision makers. Table 10.1 (overleaf) summarises the different categories discussed.

10.1 LEGISLATION

Legislation is undoubtedly the primary driver of change in the property industry. Voluntary action on a handful of showcase buildings will show what is possible but will not compel the majority to follow suit. Building regulations set the minimum legal requirements for energy efficiency in new buildings and major refurbishment (refer to Chapter 6). The regular and consistent updating of these regulations drives

	Category	Comments
1	Legislation	More stringent building regulations, the requirement to obtain minimum energy ratings for sale/lease of office buildings and mandatory reporting of energy performance will influence the value of existing buildings as well as the cost of new buildings and refurbishments.
2	Government incentives	Financial benefits can include direct payments (e.g. grants, feed-in tariffs), low interest green loans, enhanced capital tax allowances, reduced business rates and property tax relief. Faster planning approvals and density bonuses can also provide financial incentives to build greener.
3	Cost of occupancy	Rising energy costs and carbon taxes will increase the cost of occupying a building. A 25% reduction in energy consumption in a typical 10,000 m^2 air conditioned office building can deliver savings of £7/m^2. Assuming that energy costs increase by 5% per annum this is £0.9 million over 10 years.
4	Cost of occupants	People are by far the largest annual cost in an office building, and also have a significant influence on energy consumption. A green office building in London, which contributes to improving the occupant's productivity by 1%, can deliver annual cost savings of £40/m^2 (more than the total cost of energy). This equates to £4.8 million over 10 years in a 10,000 m^2 building with 750 people.
5	Brand	A trusted brand has value, although this is difficult to quantify. Brand is important to developers, designers, contractors, landlords and employers (tenants).
6	Tenant requirements	Most large corporate and government tenants have set sustainability and energy targets for the properties they build, purchase or lease. Whether they enforce these when making decisions on property is open to debate.
7	Building value	The amount, if any, of increased financial value in sustainable buildings (the 'green premium') is not yet proven. However, there appears to be broad agreement in the UK property industry that poorly performing buildings will have lower value (a 'brown discount') compared to those built to more stringent energy standards.
8	Business security	Will the building be adaptable to a changing climate and does it rely on cheap energy to be affordable to occupy?
9	Ethical investment	This is still a relatively minor driver in the property industry – but is its time coming?

Table 10.1 Summary of issues to consider in a business case for a low carbon building

efficiency improvements in design and construction, as the supply chain seeks to gain competitive advantage under the new rules by finding ways to comply for the lowest cost.

Until recently, most energy efficiency legislation related primarily to new buildings, but legislators are increasingly focusing on improving the performance of existing buildings. For example, in September 2012 the European Parliament voted to introduce new energy efficiency policies that will require all large businesses to undertake energy audits every 4 years and for central governments to renovate 3% of the total floor area of their buildings each year.[1]

Minimum energy efficiency requirements for existing buildings are being introduced in the UK. From 2018 onwards it is proposed that it will not be possible to lease office buildings which have an Energy Performance Certificate (EPC) rating of F or G.[2] It is possible that more than 20% of existing UK office stock will require upgrading to meet this rating requirement. The business case for the purchase or refurbishment of existing office buildings will need to consider the cost/benefit of improving a building to meet current or future energy efficiency standards.

'If you show me yours then I'll show you mine!'

Legislation does not have to define minimum standards to be an effective tool for change. Making it mandatory to report and publically display the annual energy consumption of individual buildings, thereby making actual energy performance visible and comparable, will provide motivation to improve performance. Reputation is important to most businesses. Recent activity in this area includes the following:

- In Australia, the mandatory disclosure of NABERS Base Building Energy ratings on the sale or lease of office buildings over 2,000 m² was introduced in 2011.[3]
- In New York City, Local Law 84, passed in 2009, mandates that all privately owned properties with individual buildings over 50,000 square feet (4,650 m²) or multiple buildings with a combined square footage over 100,000 square feet (9,300 m²) annually measure and report their energy and water use. In 2011, this included 167 million m² of property.
- The UK Government committed to making Display Energy Certificates (DECs) mandatory in the UK commercial office sector from October 2012 but subsequently failed to legislate for this despite widespread support from industry.[4] This is a major setback to encouraging landlords and tenants in the UK to reduce actual energy consumption.

At the Rio+20 summit in June 2012 the governments of the world committed to 'encouraging companies to consider' integrating sustainability into their reporting cycle.[5] While this is not exactly a call to arms, it at least acknowledges the importance of corporate sustainability reporting, particularly by large companies, as part of a sustainable future. Recent examples of mandatory corporate reporting include:

- The *Carbon Reduction Commitment – Energy Efficiency Scheme* requires UK companies and government departments with electricity consumption greater than 6,000 MWh a year to report the total carbon emissions from their combined building portfolio annually. The organisations have to purchase carbon allowances to match their emissions (effectively a carbon tax).

- All businesses listed on the Main Market of the London Stock Exchange will have to report their levels of greenhouse gas emissions from the start of April 2013.[6]
- Since 2009, it is mandatory for the 1,100 largest Danish companies, investors and state-owned companies to include information on Corporate Social Responsibility (CSR) in their annual financial reports.[7]

The trend is clear. Legislation will become increasingly tougher as governments seek to reduce their countries' energy consumption and CO_2 emissions. Building owners and developers need to understand the new and future rules to ensure that their buildings retain value – refer to Section 10.7 on Building Value.

10.2 GOVERNMENT INCENTIVES

After the stick of legislation comes the carrot of incentives. These can usually be split into two categories, planning and financial, and may be applied at a local, state or national level. It is not practical to list individual incentives here, because there are so many and they can be introduced, modified and withdrawn very rapidly. Table 10.2 summarises the types of incentives that might be available (refer to Appendix L for further discussion on these).

Type of incentive	Potential benefit
Faster planning approvals	Time is money – reduced costs in planning stage and ability to start construction sooner.
Planning density bonus	Allowing increased plot to floor area ratio or taller buildings on a site.
Business rates and property tax relief	Reduced annual costs through tax or rates reduction.
Capital allowances	Faster depreciation of energy efficiency equipment provides a net present cost benefit.
Loans for green retrofits	Ability to access low-interest loans and use energy savings to pay off the loan.
Renewable energy payments	Feed-in tariffs and other payments for the generation of renewable energy, typically over a 10- to 20-year period.
Grants and other incentives	Can include subsidies on products, matched funding for green initiatives and old equipment scrapage schemes.

Table 10.2 Examples of potential government incentives available for greening buildings

10.3 COST OF OCCUPANCY

The cost of occupancy of an office building includes:

- rent
- business rates/property taxes
- energy consumption
- landlord service charges – for maintenance, repair, management and services.

Figure 10.1 shows the typical breakdown of costs in a London office and a typical office outside London (refer to Appendix L for data used). The salary costs of occupants are discussed in the next section.

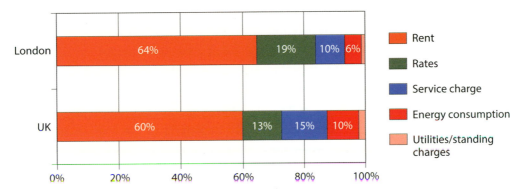

Fig 10.1 Typical breakdown of total cost of occupancy in UK offices

The era of cheap energy is almost over. The global demand for energy is increasing, fossil fuels are becoming more difficult (and costly) to extract, and the energy distribution infrastructure in many countries requires significant investment. This suggests that energy prices will continue to steadily increase above the rate of inflation, as they have done in recent years.[8]

The annual energy consumption cost (excluding demand charges) of a typical 10,000 m² air conditioned office building in the UK in 2012 was around £270,000.[9] If energy prices increase at 5% per annum then over a 10-year period the total energy cost will be almost £3.4 million. A 25% reduction in energy consumption in year 1 would save £840,000 over 10 years.

A number of countries have implemented carbon taxes, or energy taxes that are related to the carbon content of energy.[10] A carbon tax of £12/tCO_2 adds £17,000 (6%) a year to the annual energy cost of a typical 10,000 m² air conditioned office building in the UK. Assuming that the tax increases by 5% a year (to £19/tCO_2 in 2022) then the 10-year cost of the tax is £215,000. A 25% reduction in energy consumption in year 1 would save £54,000 in this tax over 10 years.

Simple low carbon buildings should, in theory, have lower landlord service charges as they will be easier to maintain and manage. Highly complex control systems can, conversely, see an increase in service charges, offsetting some of the potential energy cost savings.[11] This should be considered when developing both the business plan and the design strategy.

DO GREEN BUILDINGS HAVE HIGHER RENTS?

A study for RICS[12] in March 2012 of the London office market between 2000 and 2009 observed that 'the expanding supply of green buildings within a given London neighbourhood had a positive impact on rents and prices in general'. Other empirical studies in the USA and Australia have attempted to quantify rental increases for different rating levels using Green Star, NABERS, LEED and Energy Star.[13] These studies suggest that certified green buildings appear to attract higher rents. But is the increased rental due to the green label, or because they are higher grade offices which attract more rent anyway, and can consequently afford the extra cost of green certification?

The main problem with the studies to date relates to the small sample sizes and potentially unreliable results. Current thinking acknowledges that in order for a building to be recognised as a 'prime' building, it needs to have a green label. Anecdotal reports from market practitioners indicate that they are beginning to see a rental pricing differential between green and non-green commercial properties which correlates to the difference between prime and non-prime buildings.[14]

Further research is required to quantify whether a low energy building, by virtue of lower energy costs and brand/CSR benefits, will attract a higher rent.

10.4 COST OF OCCUPANTS

Energy is a relatively small component of the total cost of a business occupying an office building (it can be a much more significant proportion in the retail and industrial sectors). This is why legislation is required to make energy more visible to Chief Financial Officers. By far the largest business cost in an office building is the people. The average UK salary outside London is around £24,000 which increases to £43,000 in London.[15] Figure 10.2 shows the cost of people compared to the typical cost of occupancy in London. The percentage split is similar outside London (refer to Appendix L for assumptions).

The quality of a building's internal environment can influence productivity but, as there are so many other factors (work/life balance, sense of achievement, quality of bosses), it is difficult to measure accurately and then attribute to specific features of a building. Methods of measuring productivity include reduction in short-term sick leave and improvements in quality or quantity of specific tasks. Various studies have

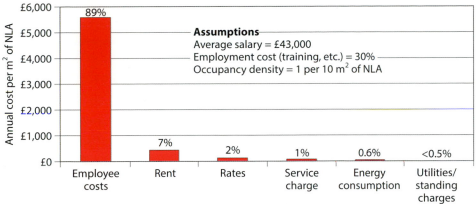

Fig 10.2 Typical business costs of an office building in London

shown the impact that ventilation rates, air quality, temperature control and quality of light and views can have on productivity.[16]

A 1% improvement in staff productivity in London is equivalent to £40/m² per year, which is more than the total cost of energy. In a 10,000 m² office with 750 occupants this equates to £4.8 million over 10 years. While more research is required to quantify long-term productivity gains in greener buildings (and the reasons for these), the business case for delivering modest improvements is certainly compelling.

PRODUCTIVITY IN BUILDINGS: THE KILLER VARIABLES

The Usable Buildings Trust have identified a number of key issues related to productivity in buildings.[17] These include :

- productivity of building occupants can only be estimated practically by subjective means
- believable data on perceived productivity is hard to find – be suspicious of inflated claims
- what exists is usually not put into a context which designers, building managers and corporate decision-makers can easily understand
- thermal discomfort is usually the number one productivity killer
- people are more likely to be tolerant when they have more control, even if the conditions themselves are not measurably better
- buildings that deliver rapid response to need, either through the physical design or the management system, are usually better
- irrelevant noise is increasingly significant
- green buildings can often make the mistake of introducing too much unwanted complication
- complexity often ends up with systems defaulting to the 'least worst' for everyone
- the more workgroup boundaries 'map' onto building services zones the better
- make design intent clear – people forgive faults if they know how things are supposed to work.

10.5 BRAND

A UN Global Compact–Accenture survey[18] of 766 CEOs in 2010 identified that 'demonstrating a visible and authentic commitment to sustainability is especially important to CEOs because it is part of an urgent need to regain and build trust from the public and other key stakeholders, such as consumers and governments'. Some 72% identified strengthening brand, trust and reputation as the strongest motivators for taking action on sustainability issues. Revenue growth and cost reduction was second with 44%.

A survey by Gensler[19] in 2006 showed that, of the factors most likely to make businesses consider energy efficiency when procuring buildings, brand differentiation scored only 2% (with energy costs, tax incentives and legislation all scoring over 30%). There appears to be a disconnect between the views of CEOs and the individuals making decisions about property. This will not be bridged until sustainability becomes embedded in individual performance frameworks for managers across organisations, which may take some time.

Table 10.3 provides examples of the potential benefits of a credible brand in sustainability for different types of organisation.

Organisation	Potential benefit to brand
Developers	Local authorities, by granting planning permission, give developers a 'licence to trade' and need to be able to trust the developer to deliver. The developer's sustainability credentials and brand are an increasingly important consideration when deciding whether to allow a development to proceed, or whether the council will partner with the developer on projects.
Landlords	A landlord who can demonstrate that they work collaboratively with their tenants to deliver more productive workplaces, lower energy costs and sustainability initiatives should be more attractive to potential and existing tenants. This does, however, rely on estate agents and tenants' representatives clearly understanding the benefits of greener buildings.
Tenants (employers)	In 2007, prior to the global downturn in 2008, a survey of college graduates in the USA suggested that 80% were interested in a job that has a positive impact on the environment and 92% would chose to work for an environmentally friendly company.[20] Tenants seeking to attract the best talent will find it harder to demonstrate sustainability credentials in high energy consuming buildings (which is one reason why the mandatory public display of energy performance will motivate both landlords and tenants to act).
Designers and contractors	It is rare that a new building project brief does not contain the words 'demonstrate your environmental credentials', or words to that effect, somewhere in the selection criteria. Designers and contractors who can demonstrate a track record in the cost effective delivery of low carbon buildings stand a better chance of being invited to tender and subsequently winning the work.

Table 10.3 Brand benefits of sustainability in different organisations

10.6 TENANT REQUIREMENTS

In the RICS report *Supply, Demand and the Value of Green Buildings* published in 2012,[21] CBRE reports that '58% of tenants find energy efficiency essential and 50% find green attributes essential. Anecdotally, the move of tenants towards green real estate is due to enhanced reputation benefits, corporate social responsibility mandates and employee productivity. Shifting tenant preferences suggests tenants are using the buildings they occupy to communicate their corporate vision to shareholders and employees.'

Many large corporate companies and government departments set energy and sustainability targets and requirements for the commercial offices they lease. This can include minimum energy ratings (e.g. EPC, Energy Star, NABERS) and green building ratings (e.g. BREEAM, LEED, Green Star). While location, quality, availability, suitability and affordability will usually always take precedence in the decision making process, if the building is not seen to be green it may be less likely to be shortlisted and then chosen compared to a similar building which has certification. In a competitive market this could mean missing out on a major tenant or taking longer to lease the building.

That is the theory. The reality is that, over the last ten years, very few prospective tenants (public or private) have considered energy performance prior to signing leases.[22] It is not high on their list of business priorities. Would this change if energy performance was displayed prominently in the foyer, shown in corporate reports and made freely accessible to the media?

The willingness of landlords and/or tenants to enter into Green Leases is another consideration. These were supported by the Federal Government in Australia as a means to establish regular dialogue and cooperation between landlord and government tenants to reduce the energy consumption of office buildings. How effectively they are being implemented in practice is unclear. Other countries have considered the idea, but they have not yet been widely adopted. Appendix L provides further details.

10.7 BUILDING VALUE

Investment in reducing energy consumption in buildings is usually made on the basis that the capital cost will be paid back over a period of time (the payback period) through energy cost savings. While this makes good business sense for owner-occupiers and landlord base building services, if the cost benefit of a landlord's investment in energy savings goes directly to the tenant then it may be difficult to justify unless:

- they can charge a higher rent
- they are trying to attract, or retain, an energy-conscious tenant
- the energy improvements increase the value of the building.

The last item is analogous to buying shares where the dividend (energy cost savings) goes to a third party (the tenant), and the benefit to the purchaser (building owner) is the increase in share value (capital value of the building). But is there any evidence that energy efficient or greener buildings have a higher value?

There are two schools of thought on building value. The first assumes that low carbon, environmentally friendly buildings (the high achievers) are worth more than standard buildings and attract a *green premium*.[23] The alternative view is that green buildings will hold their value, but that there is no compelling evidence that such a premium exists, and instead there is a *brown discount*. This assumes that poorly performing energy-guzzling buildings (the delinquents) will be worth less in the future.

The reasoning for the *brown discount* is that the introduction of minimum energy requirements for existing buildings, and the potential mandatory display of actual energy performance, will speed up the rate of obsolescence of poorly performing buildings. They will either attract lower rents, reducing their value, or will require costly intervention to bring them up to the prevailing green standards. It is likely that many portfolio owners will seek to dispose of inefficient stock and refurbish those buildings which can be cost effectively upgraded.

There is clearly a need for more sophisticated analysis when looking at sustainability and building valuation, due to the complex and varying factors influencing the value of buildings. Whether you pay more for good or less for bad, the future is clear, all other things being equal, low carbon buildings should be worth more than high carbon buildings.

10.8 FUTURE BUSINESS SECURITY

In the UN Global Compact–Accenture CEO survey in 2010,[24] 93% of CEOs considered sustainability as important to their company's future. Two critical development issues that CEOs identified for the future success of their business were:

- education (72%) – the failure of education systems, talent pipelines and the capabilities of future leaders to manage sustainability
- climate change (66%) – the need to reduce greenhouse gas emissions and adapt to a changing climate.

The survey identified three key ways in which approaches and strategies issues are shifting:

- the consumer is (or will be) king
- technology and innovation are important
- collaboration is critical.

In 2012, the report *Insights into Climate Change Adaptation by UK Companies*[25] found that 80% of FTSE 100 companies surveyed identify substantial risks to their business from climate change, but only 46% have included adaptation plans in their business strategies.

Two issues which may directly impact on new and existing buildings in the future are:

- the ability to adapt to a changing climate – will this affect the insurability of assets less resilient to extreme weather events? Will poorly insulated air conditioned glass boxes be habitable in the future without major renovation or large energy bills?[26]
- security of energy supply – as global demand for energy increases, affordable fossil fuel reserves reduce and old energy infrastructure starts to fail, then will a reliable supply of energy always be available, and how useable is a building under such a scenario?[27]

10.9 ETHICAL INVESTMENT?

Ethics are moral guidelines which govern good behaviour. Behaving ethically in business is widely regarded as good business practice:

- 'A business which makes nothing but money is a poor kind of business' – Henry Ford
- 'Being good is good business' – Anita Roddick.

Ethical principles and standards in business define acceptable conduct and underpin how management make decisions. This is a complex issue – in most issues of business ethics, ideal moral principles may be tempered by economic viability.[28]

In 2012 ethical investment funds accounted for around 1.2% of funds under management in the UK.[29] This is consequently a relatively small player in the property industry. A report in 2010 by the Institutional Investors Group on Climate Change,[30] which includes some of the largest pension funds and asset managers in Europe, representing assets exceeding €5 trillion, stated:

> the belief is growing that, over time, more environmentally conscious buildings will experience higher net income growth and be viewed as lower risk and thereby deliver higher returns. If environmental issues are set to affect the current and future value and performance of property assets, then the environmental performance of property assets must be seen as a fiduciary as well as a social responsibility for pension funds.

The report poses the questions that pension funds should ask regarding the environmental performance of buildings and portfolios. The key word here is 'should' as there is little evidence to suggest that the investment decisions of pension funds are currently driving the commercial property industry to significantly reduce energy and carbon – although this may change in the future.

The UN Global Compact–Accenture survey noted that 86% of CEOs see 'accurate valuation by investors of sustainability in long-term investments' as important to reaching a tipping point in sustainability. Attracting ethical investment is not yet a major driver for greening the property industry – but its time appears to be coming.

10.10 SUMMARY

While many will consider investing in low carbon buildings a no-brainer, not much happens without either a big stick (legislation) or a suitable carrot (financial benefit and corporate reputation). This chapter has outlined some of the direct and indirect financial benefits that might be used in a business case to justify investing in low carbon buildings, either new or refurbished. Which ones apply will depend on who is preparing the business case and who the decision makers are – refer to Figure 10.3.

The business case could be a detailed cost benefit analysis of a lighting upgrade made by the facility manager in a building,[31] or it could be a strategic business case regarding the long-term composition of an international property portfolio. Whatever the project, it should be possible to make a compelling business case for investing in energy and carbon reduction in buildings – it is just a case of putting the right ingredients together.

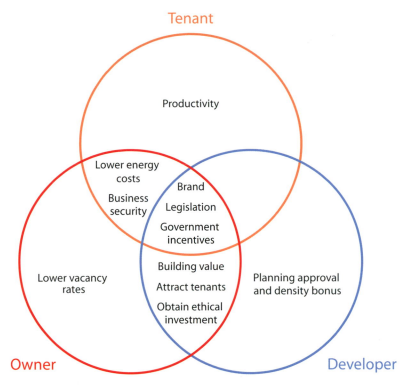

Fig 10.3 **Summary of business case issues for tenants, developers and building owners**

THE COST OF BUILDING GREEN

This chapter has discussed the potential benefits of greener buildings but not the cost. There is a perception amongst some industry professionals that building green increases costs by 10 to 20%.[32] This can lead to low carbon solutions being prematurely dismissed as 'too expensive' without taking time at the start of a project to develop options further and test the cost impacts properly. Various studies show that the actual costs range between −0.4 and 12.5%. Changing the misconception that we can't afford to go green is essential to delivering low carbon buildings.

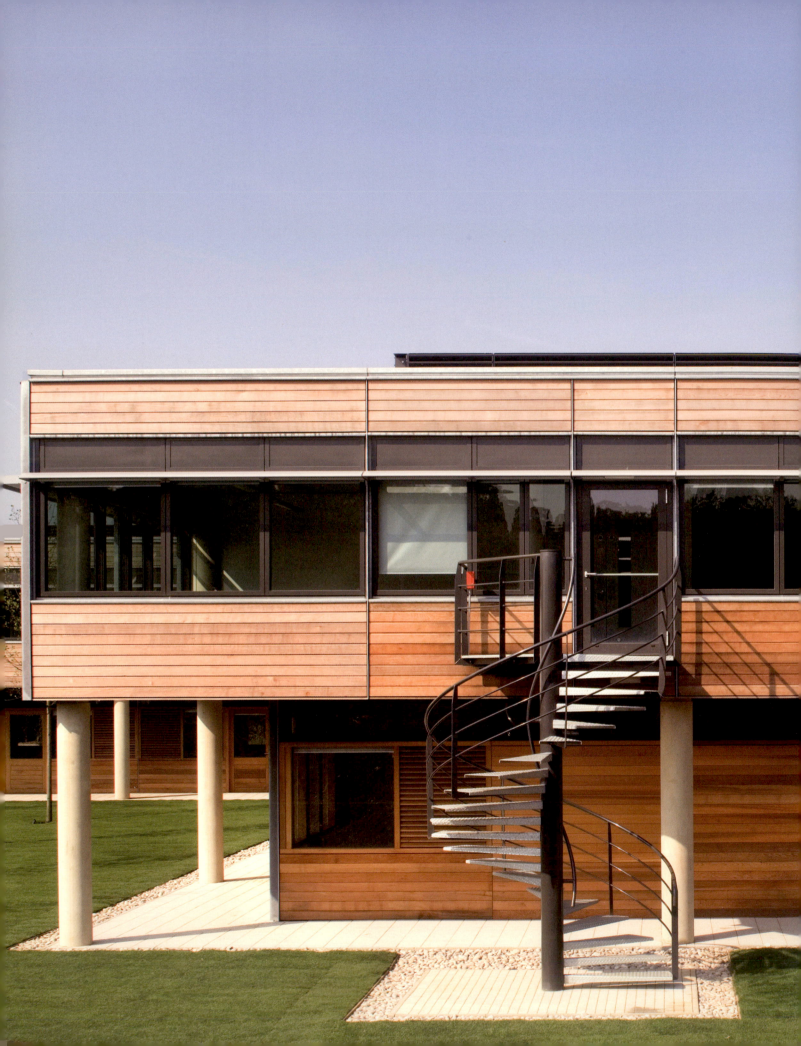

In conclusion

This book has attempted to do two things: to put the whole carbon footprint of office buildings into perspective, and to identify practical opportunities to reduce energy consumption and CO_2e emissions. The carbon footprint, which can also be a reasonable proxy for energy resource consumption, comprises the CO_2e emissions due to operating, embodied and transport energy.

Energy consumption is not visible in most office buildings or board rooms. Until government and the property sector acknowledge that actual performance is more important than good intentions (design ratings), make energy data publically available, and then invest in behavioural change and efficient technologies, significant energy and carbon reduction in office buildings is likely to remain elusive. Tougher legislation, clearer incentives and mechanisms for landlords and tenants to work closely together are needed.

Building design doesn't need a radical overhaul – just a healthy dose of common sense and the application of good design principles. Architects need to rethink façade design to increase useful daylight and thermal comfort, and reduce heat losses in winter and solar gains in summer. Engineers need to design for low annual energy consumption (i.e. efficient operation every day) and not just to meet peak loads which only occur on a handful of days each year. Facility managers need to better understand how to drive their buildings efficiently, which is often easier if the controls are not too complicated.

Renewable energy systems in buildings can only practically contribute between 5 and 10% of CO_2e reduction, and so providing simple mechanisms to allow building owners and occupants to invest in more cost effective large scale off-site renewable energy generation is necessary.

Embodied carbon is getting a lot of attention, but in most office buildings it is still a relatively small component of the whole carbon footprint. It provides a reasonable proxy for material resource efficiency, but more research is required to obtain better data on the embodied carbon of materials, products and buildings. Designers and purchasers can help to drive embodied energy and carbon reduction in the supply chain by using purchasing power to favour lower carbon products.

The location of an office building has a surprisingly large impact on the whole carbon footprint, which in some cases can be greater than the operating and embodied carbon combined. This is another topic warranting further research, in particular how building owners and employers can encourage people to use greener modes of transport.

The book has focused on individual buildings, but to deliver a low carbon city will require some joined up government and industry thinking. Imagine if the following scenario was to occur in a city near you sometime in the not too distant future.

Natural gas has run out, or has become prohibitively expensive and unreliable to source, and buildings rely more on electricity and district heating systems for heat instead of gas boilers.

Combustion engines are banned in city centres and only electric or hydrogen powered vehicles are permitted to enter, making the streets much quieter and reducing air pollution. At the same time planning rules require that hard surfaces be treated to reduce the heat island effect,[1] including planting green roofs, lowering the local air temperature by a degree or so on hot summer days.

Legislation requiring energy efficient IT systems slashes server energy consumption and LED lighting technology has made fluorescents obsolete. The reduction in internal heat loads, external temperatures, noise and air pollution leads to a rediscovery of openable windows in city centres!

Building regulations get tougher and target energy consumption as well as energy efficiency. It becomes a requirement to be able to use natural ventilation and daylight effectively in new buildings, mainly by limiting the depth of floor plates to around 16 m. Procurement processes focus on collaboration instead of confrontation, reducing construction costs and leading to thousands of lawyers retraining to use their skills to benefit society.

Legislation, triggered on the sale or rent of existing buildings, requires substantial improvements to the thermal performance of the fabric, retrofitting energy efficient lighting and HVAC systems, and giving occupants access to natural ventilation whenever practical.

Energy tariff structures are turned upside down. Adopting a similar approach to income tax, energy consumption is split into bands, with unit rates (£ per kWh) increasing as consumption increases (currently energy pricing works the other way round – the more you use the cheaper the rate). Users can also negotiate discounted rates by agreeing to limit their peak demand (kW) and pay penalties if they exceed this (similar to bank charges for exceeding agreed overdraft limits).

Behavioural change programmes start to pay off, with people allowed to dress appropriately to suit the seasons, and getting into the habit of switching stuff off when it is not needed. Many organisations start to link energy cost savings to staff bonuses.[2] The cost and carbon emissions of the landlord's and tenant's annual energy consumption is prominently displayed in the foyer of every commercial building and available on Google maps.

While this probably represents an overly simplistic solution to a complex problem, it is certainly achievable (perhaps with the exception of the lawyers). The technologies needed already exist and market forces will see further efficiency gains while costs reduce significantly. For example, LED office lighting will very quickly become affordable if the LED TV industry is any indicator of the effect of global competition.[3] It wasn't many years ago that compact fluorescents were completely unaffordable to households.

The property industry has the capacity to make radical changes, but currently does not have a compelling need to do so. The key catalyst required is political will. If government places levers in the right places then, after the initial and inevitable complaints of unaffordability, property and construction companies will simply get on with developing the solutions to give them a competitive advantage. However, to encourage the investment needed, the rules have to be both consistent (joined up thinking across government departments) and long term (to not change suddenly on a political whim). Unfortunately, this is where it all starts to go wrong. Sensationalist headlines in the media about the cost of going green do not encourage politicians to think beyond the next election cycle.

Informing both government and the media of the need for the right legislation, and the long-term cost benefits of this, is probably as important in the delivery of significant change as developing the actual solutions to deliver energy and carbon savings in buildings. Hopefully, this book will contribute positively to all of these aspects.

Savings by Fiona MacKenzie, IHS BRE Press, 2010.

20 The World Green Building Council website www.worldgbc.org listed 91 councils in September 2012: 26 established, 12 emerging, 19 associated and 34 prospective.

21 Refer to **Appendix A** for an overview of the science of climate change and **Appendix B** for $kgCO_2e$ emission factors for different fuels.

22 **Appendix B** provides grid electricity emission factors for different countries and includes an explanation for the $0.6\ kgCO_2e/kWh$ factor adopted in this book.

23 UK consumption emissions are 34% higher than UK production emissions with Germany (29%), Japan (19%) and the USA (13%) also big importers. Developing countries are generally net exporters of CO_2 emissions. For example, in 2004 China exported 23% of all its domestically produced CO_2. *International Carbon Flows: Global Flows*, Carbon Trust, 2011, CTC795. www.carbontrust.com/our-clients/i/international-carbon-flows.

24 *Consumption-Based Emissions Reporting*, twelfth report of session 2010–12, volume 1, Energy & Climate Change Committee (published 18 April 2013). The report recommended exploring options to incorporate consumption-based emissions data into the policy making process and also noted that:
- the fall in the UK's emissions over the last 20 years was primarily due to switching from coal to gas-fired electricity generation and not due to the government's climate policy
- the 9% fall in the UK's consumption-based emissions between 2008 and 2009 was primarily a result of the economic downturn, rather than of the UK's policies to reduce greenhouse gas emissions. Discounting the effects of the recession, the UK's consumption-based emissions have been on an upward trend since 1990

- electricity intensive industries should not receive energy subsidies unless they commit to energy efficiency improvements, as their investment decisions are not currently being driven by government climate policy but by volatility in the fossil fuel market.

25 Figure 1.4 is sourced from Davis, S.J., Peters, G.P. and Caldeira, K. (2011) *The Supply Chain of CO$_2$ Emissions*, PNAS. www.pnas.org/cgi/doi/10.1073/pnas.1107409108. Data for individual countries can be obtained from http://supplychainco2.stanford.edu/graphics.html.

26 Refer to **Appendix L** for further information on corporate reporting.

27 Primary energy factors for the UK are taken from the UK Passivhaus calculator (2007), UK Standard Assessment Procedure (SAP) 2009 and the US Energy Star protocols. Refer to **Appendix A** for more details. Primary energy factors are often used in Europe instead of CO_2 due to the wide differences in grid electricity emission factors, from $0.06\ kgCO_2/kWh$ in Sweden to $0.97\ kgCO_2/kWh$ in Greece. Refer to **Appendix B** for full list of CO_2e emission factors.

28 The domestic tariffs are taken from the author's electricity and gas bills in October 2012. Refer to Chapter 7 for the commercial tariffs used in the renewable energy system calculations.

29 The UK's Display Energy Certificate, which benchmarks energy performance, is based on $kgCO_2/m^2$ and not kWh/m^2 because 'the UK has decided that the common unit should be CO_2 emissions, since this is a key driver for energy policy'. *Improving the Energy Efficiency of our Buildings: A guide to Display Energy Certificates and Advisory Reports for Public Buildings*, Department for Communities and Local Government, May 2008.

The NABERS Energy rating tool in Australia also uses $kgCO_2/m^2$ as the benchmark. The US Energy Star system uses primary energy. Refer to Appendix C for more details on these rating tools.

30 BOGOF means 'buy one get one free'. Reducing CO_2e emissions, while ensuring security and affordability of supply is known as the 'energy trilemma'.

CHAPTER 2
How much energy do buildings use?

All websites accessed 30 January 2013 unless noted otherwise.

1   Refer to Chapter 10 for comparison of salary, rates, rent, service charges and energy bills in London and the UK as a whole. Energy represents between 6% and 11% of the cost of office occupancy and less than 1% if the cost of people (salaries) is included.

2   These rating tools benchmark the energy performance of buildings or occupants using 12 months of metered energy consumption. Refer to **Appendix C** for further details.

3   For further information on the EU Energy Performance in Buildings Directive, including the Nearly Zero Energy Building requirements, refer to **Appendix L**.

4   For background and definition of a 'zero carbon home' in the UK refer to **Appendix L**.

5   According to the British Council for Offices' *Occupier Density Study Summary Report* (June 2009), the average occupancy density in UK offices in 2008 was around one person per 12 m² of Net Internal Area. Using a factor of 1.25 to convert to GIA this gives 1 per 15 m². Refer to **Appendix D** for further details.

6   Refer to **Appendix C** for breakdown of calculations and assumptions made.

7   The Passivhaus standard was developed in Germany in the early 1990s for housing, but has subsequently been applied to offices (refer to www.passivhaus.org.uk). It requires a highly insulated, well-sealed building fabric, which then minimises the need for heating. Ducted fresh air with heat recovery is usually provided, and cooling is typically via natural ventilation. The heating load must be less than 10 W/m² or the annual heating and cooling energy demand combined must be less than 15 kWh/m². The primary energy limit is 120 kWh/m² which equates to 44 kWh/m² of electricity (26.5 kgCO₂e/m²). The 'lowest energy office' could achieve this with 50% of the roof covered with PV panels provided it was no more than five storeys tall (refer to Figure 2.2).

8   Energy audits undertaken by the author of four UK office buildings in 2011 suggest that server rooms can account for between 30 and 40% of the tenant's light and power energy consumption – around 20% of the total operating CO_2e emissions of the building. Unfortunately, they are rarely submetered. **Appendix H** provides more details of server room energy.

9   The annual output from the PV system is 117 kWh/m² of panel. Refer to **Appendix C** for calculations. Further details on outputs and cost/benefit of PV systems are discussed in Chapter 7.

10 Thermal comfort is discussed further in Chapter 6 and in **Information Paper 33 – Productivity in office buildings.**

11 *Energy benchmarks – TM46:2008* published by CIBSE provides the benchmarks used for DECs in England, Wales and Northern Ireland and explains the approach to their development and use. The energy benchmark for offices is 95 kWh/m² for electricity and 120 kWh/m² for thermal (gas). Using this book's emission factors (kgCO₂e/kWh) of 0.6 for electricity and 0.2 for gas gives a CO_2e benchmark of 81 kgCO₂e/m². The emission factors used in the DEC rating tool and CIBSE guide are 0.551 and 0.190 respectively, giving a benchmark of 75 kgCO₂/m². The DEC emission factors are also different from other UK Government factors for EPCs, building regulations and corporate reporting.

13 Refer to **Information Paper 12 – Embodied carbon case studies for office buildings** for a summary of Stanhope ECO_2 fit-out data including conversion to GIA.

14 *Cutting Embodied Carbon in Construction Projects*, a WRAP information sheet for construction clients and designers. www.wrap.org.uk/sites/files/wrap/FINAL%20PRO095-009%20Embodied%20Carbon%20Annex.pdf.

15 *The Green Guide to Specification*, 3rd edition, by Anderson, J., Shiers, D. and Sinclair, M., published by Blackwell Science, Oxford, 2002. The Green Guide ratings for all the elements used in BREEAM can now be found on line at www.bre.co.uk/greenguide.

16 Developed by BRE, an Ecopoint is a single score that measures the total environmental impact of a product or process as a proportion of the overall impact occurring in Europe. 100 Ecopoints is equivalent to the impact of a European citizen over the course of 1 year. The points are determined by multiplying Environmental Profiles data for 13 impacts by weightings (which were determined via a consensus-based research programme). The impacts are: climate change, fossil fuel depletion, ozone depletion, freight transport, human toxicity to air, human toxicity to water, waste disposal, water extraction, acid deposition, ecotoxicity, eutrophication, summer smog and minerals extraction.

17 'Assessing embodied energy of building structural elements', Vukotic, L., Fenner, R. and Symons, K. *Proceedings of the ICE – Engineering Sustainability*, Vol. 163, No. 3, Sept. 2010, pp. 147–58.

18 In November 2012, WRAP and UK Green Building Council commissioned a study to develop a freely available database for the embodied carbon of buildings. One stated aim was that, if the dataset became large and robust enough, then ECO_2 benchmarks for buildings could be developed. Such benchmarks would need to reflect the standards/methodologies used, the ECO_2 factors applied and the assumptions made for end of life.

19 The base case operating energy of $100 \ kgCO_2e/m^2$ is the author's assumed benchmark for a typical commercial office building in the UK (refer to Chapter 2). This is based on actual consumption for the whole building. The EU standard EN 15978 states that design or actual energy consumption can be used, but that small power should not be included when comparing to embodied carbon. If small power was excluded it would reduce the operating energy figure to around $75 \ kgCO_2e/m^2$. This increases the proportion of initial construction ECO_2 from 12% to 15% (equivalent to 10 years of operating energy) for the base case. The embodied carbon of the small power equipment (e.g. PC, fridges, etc.) would ideally have been included in the assessment in this book but there is insufficient data available.

20 The Target Emission Rate (TER) for a new office building to Part L 2010 building regulations is around $25 \ kgCO_2e/m^2$ (refer Figure 6.1 in Chapter 6). If the initial embodied carbon is $700 \ kgCO2e/m^2$ then this is equivalent to the TER x 28 years.

   The proposition sometimes espoused, that when new buildings become zero carbon (TER = $0 \ kgCO_2e/m^2$) then embodied carbon will account for 100% of the carbon footprint, does not really stand up to any kind of scrutiny. This is because, in real life, buildings are not zero carbon.

21 In Hong Kong, Life Cycle Assessment (including embodied carbon) is required to be undertaken on all government projects for building approval, although no minimum standards are set. In June 2011, the UK Government prepared a Low Carbon Construction Action Plan, which recommended that embodied carbon should be considered as well as operating carbon, and that industry should agree a standard method of measurement. It noted

that the enthusiasm to develop industry approaches to measuring embodied carbon had 'resulted in multiple standards and methodologies creating confusion'. www.bis.gov.uk/assets/BISCore/business-sectors/docs/l/11-976-low-carbon-construction-action-plan.pdf. Refer also to note 18 for the potential development of ECO_2 benchmarks in the UK.

22 Refer to **Information Paper 15 – Whole carbon footprint in rating tools** for further details.

CHAPTER 4
Transport carbon

All websites accessed 30 January 2013 unless noted otherwise.

1   The *Personal Travel Factsheet: Commuting and Business Travel* published by National Statistics and the Department for Transport and in April 2011 notes that commuting accounts for 15% of the number of all trips, and business trips account for 3% of trips. Commuting and business trips tend to be longer than other trips (e.g. going shopping) and so account for a greater proportion of total distance travelled (19% and 8% respectively).

2   Taken from the data tables with the *2011 UK Greenhouse Gas Emissions: Final Figures*, a statistical release by the Department of Energy and Climate Change dated 5 February 2013. www.gov.uk/government/organisations/department-of-energy-climate-change/series/uk-greenhouse-gas-emissions.

3   Data from Table 2.3 in the *Energy Consumption in the United Kingdom – Transport Data Tables – 2012 update* by the Department of Energy and Climate Change. www.gov.uk/government/organisations/department-of-energy-climate-change/series/energy-consumption-in-the-uk.

4   Data from Table 2.7 – refer to note 3.

5   The *Personal Travel Factsheet: Commuting and Business Travel* published by the Department for Transport and Office of National Statistics (April 2011) noted that the mode of transport varies depending on distance to place of work with the proportion of commuting trips by surface rail increasing with trip length.

6   Refer to **Appendix F** for the data used to create Figure 4.3. This includes details of the various surveys, the analysis of the 2002 census data by Peter Wyatt of University of Reading, and the Travel Survey methodology used for all Cundall offices in 2011. It should be noted that the travel surveys use different survey techniques and different CO_2 emission factors for travel modes, which means that direct comparison between surveys is not possible. Instead, the intention is to put the $kgCO_2e$/person into perspective so that it can be compared to operating and embodied carbon.

7   *The Fourth Carbon Budget: Reducing Emissions Through the 2020s* published by the Committee on Climate Change, December 2010.

CHAPTER 5
Whole carbon footprint

1   Refer to **Appendix C** for breakdown of annual energy consumption and to **Appendix F** for commuting travel survey data in Cundall's UK offices.

2   Refer to **Information Paper 14 – Land use efficiency: city centre versus rural** for an example calculation of land area per person for a ten-storey city centre office (one person per 1.5 m²) compared to a two-storey rural office (one person per 26 m²).

3   In the example, the 10% renewables target was based on a building just achieving an assumed Part L Building Regulations 2010 Target Emissions Rate (TER) of 25 $kgCO_2$/m² – refer to **Information**

Paper 9 – Design energy rating data for a breakdown of this assumed value.

4   The benchmark for an existing building by area excludes the embodied carbon due to initial construction. The unadjusted benchmark by area from Table 5.2 is therefore $203 - 12 = 191$ kgCO$_2$e/m^2 of GIA. To convert this to an occupancy benchmark, multiply by the default occupancy of one person per 15 m^2 = 191 × 15 = 2,865 kgCO$_2$e/person.

CHAPTER 6
Ten steps to reducing energy consumption

All websites accessed 30 January 2013 unless noted otherwise.

1   Refer to Information Paper 9 – Design energy rating data for data used.

2   The UK Energy Act 2011 requires that, from 2018, all commercial buildings must have a minimum Energy Performance Certificate (EPC) rating on sale or lease – the benchmark is intended to be set at an E rating. Since 2011, disclosure of a landlord's NABERS base building energy rating (which is based on metered, not modelled, energy) is mandatory on the sale or lease of office buildings greater than 2,000 m^2 in Australia. Refer to Appendix C for further details.

3   The NABERS rating tool for office energy is based on operating energy consumption of either the base building (landlord) or a tenancy or the whole building. There is no design rating certificate, but energy modelling is used to estimate the operating energy for NABERS Energy Commitment Agreements and/or Green Star ratings. These can be downloaded from the resources page of www.nabers.gov.au. The modelling guide states that:
      'The use of a simulation as one part of determining energy performance is secondary in importance and authority to the recommendations of the NABERS Energy Independent Energy Efficiency Design Review. This is because any

realistic determination of energy performance involves a substantial amount of professional judgement about factors that are either impractical or impossible to simulate.'
In other words, common sense is more important than computers.

4   Building Regulations 2010 Approved Document L2A, clause 4.38 requires installation of energy metering systems that enable:
   - at least 90% of the annual energy consumption of each fuel to be assigned to the various end-use categories (heating, lighting, etc.). Detailed guidance on how this can be achieved is given in CIBSE TM39; and
   - the output of any renewable energy system to be separately monitored; and
   - in buildings with a total useful floor area greater than 1,000 m^2, automatic data reading and collection facilities.

5   Refer to Information Paper 16 – Heating degree days for an estimate of the gas energy savings due to changing the AHU timer clock, taking into consideration the different heating degree days before and after.

6. Lux (lumens per m^2) is a measure of the amount of light on a surface. BS12464:1 (2011) gives 500 lux as a minimum for reading tasks and 300 lux for screen based tasks, applied over a minimum task area of 0.5m x 0.5m. Refer to Appendix H for further details.

7   There is compelling evidence on the importance of daylight and views to the productivity of people in buildings. For further details refer to Information Paper 33 – Productivity in office buildings.

8   Refer to Appendix H and Information Paper 17 – Thermal comfort standards for further details on thermal comfort standards, physical factors and how the body gains and loses heat.

9   Taken from the British Council for Offices (BCO) *Guide to Specification 2009*.

10 Operative temperature is a single value to express the joint effect of air temperature and mean radiant temperature. It is calculated using a weighting that reflects the heat transfer by convection and radiation at the clothed surface of the occupant. It can be adjusted to reflect different air speeds and clothing types. Refer to CIBSE Guide A, Section 1 for further details.

11 Refer to **Appendix H** for details plus an assessment of potential energy savings due to adopting a similar strategy in an Australian city.

12 The adaptive approach to thermal comfort is based on observations (field studies not lab experiments) that people in daily life are not passive in relation to their environment. They tend to make themselves comfortable, given time and opportunity, by making adjustments (adaptations) to their clothing, activity and posture, as well as to their thermal environment. Refer to **Information Paper 17 – Thermal comfort standards** for further details.

13 This is a complex issue and difficult to quantify. The Federation of European HVAC Association (REHVA) *Guidebook No. 6* provides a rule of thumb that every temperature of 1 °C above 25 °C results in a fall off in productivity of 2%. This may be oversimplistic due to the complexity of issues affecting productivity. Refer to **Information Paper 33 – Productivity in office buildings** for more discussion on productivity due to temperature, air quality, ventilation rates and daylight.

14 The US Environmental Protection Agency (EPA) publication *The Inside Story: A Guide to Indoor Air Quality* makes reference to research findings that people spend approximately 90% of their time indoors. www.epa.gov/iaq/pubs/insidestory.html.

15 Refer to **Information Paper 18 – Types of blinds for offices** for examples.

16 'Identifying determinants of energy use in the UK non-domestic stock', Harry Bruhns, *Proceedings of the Fifth International Conference on Improving Energy Efficiency in Commercial Buildings*, Frankfurt, April 2008. Refer also to **Information Paper 10 – Area and age of UK office stock**.

17 For a list of the thermal performance requirements in UK building regulations since 1950, refer to **Appendix H**.

18 Calculation based on ECON 19 values – refer to **Information Paper 9 – Design energy rating data** for data.

19 UK, US and Australian standards and guidelines typically require between 7.5 and 10 l/s of fresh air per person in typical office environments – refer to **Information Paper 20 – Ventilation rates in offices** for more details.

20 LEED New Construction 2011, IEQ-2 awards one point for a 30% increase in fresh air above the minimum requirement of ASHRAE Standard 62.1-2007. This is approximately 11 l/s/person assuming a default value of 8.5 l/s/person. Green Star Office v3, IEQ-1 awards one to three points for 50 to 150% increase in fresh air above the minimum requirement of AS1668.2-1991. This is approximately 11.3 to 18.8 l/s/person. This can be reduced by using higher quality filters in the ventilation system.

21 The 5% rule is based on being able to provide sufficient air changes per hour to remove heat from a UK building in summer. This approach is also referenced in BREEAM 2011 (refer to **Appendix H**). **Information Paper 20 – Ventilation rates in offices – mechanical and natural** includes a comparison of the 5% rule of thumb with the CIBSE Guide AM10 calculation methodology referenced in UK Building Regulations Part F.

   Note: free area and effective ventilation area are not the same. Free area is the physical size of the opening. Effective area is determined in a test facility based on the resistance to airflow through the opening.

22 Table 6.2 of CIBSE Guide F gives internal heat loads (W/m²) in offices for different occupancy densities – refer to **Appendix H**.

23 A study of 767 fans in Sweden measured the average total efficiency at 33% (refer to **Appendix H**).

24 Refer to note 7 in Chapter 2.

25 *'The major difference between a thing that might go wrong and a thing that cannot possibly go wrong is that when a thing that cannot possibly go wrong goes wrong it usually turns out to be impossible to get at or repair.'* In *Mostly Harmless*, the fifth book of the Hitch Hiker's Guide to the Galaxy, Douglas Adams then goes on to describe the Great Ventilation and Telephone Riots of SrDt 3454 caused by the failure of the Breathe-O-Smart in-building climate control systems:

> *'The major differences from just ordinary air-conditioning were that it was thrillingly more expensive, involved a huge amount of sophisticated measuring and regulating equipment which was far better at knowing, moment by moment, what kind of air people wanted to breathe than mere people did. It also meant that, to be sure that mere people didn't muck up the sophisticated calculations which the system was making on their behalf, all the windows in the buildings were built shut. This is true.'*

The description of how it all went wrong is pretty funny but unfortunately too long to include here.

26 This data is based on ECON 19 benchmarks for a Type 3 air conditioned office building (refer to **Appendix C**). Data from the Carbon Trust (*Heating, Ventilation and Air Conditioning: Saving Energy Without Compromising Comfort*, CTV046, 2011) suggests that heating accounts for 46% of total carbon emissions from energy use in public and commercial buildings (which includes schools, police stations, offices and hospitals) with just 7% for ventilation and cooling – these are primarily older buildings with natural ventilation and radiators, and limited air conditioning.

27 Refer to **Information Paper 21 – Overview of HVAC systems in office buildings** for descriptions of different heating, cooling and ventilation systems commonly used in office buildings.

28 There are many detailed HVAC design guides available. Refer to **Appendix H**.

29 The lighting energy consumption calculated using EPC/Part L approved software for a new office is typically 10 kWh/m² and represents around 35% of the total EPC rating score of 28 kgCO$_2$e/m². From ECON 19 benchmarks (refer to **Appendix C**), lighting represents about 24% of the operating energy (if small power is included the percentage reduces further).

30 LENI is the lighting energy consumption per annum divided by the floor area, calculated in accordance with EN 15193. It is a much better measure of efficiency than W/m² (the installed power) because it takes into account the benefit of daylight and controls, to determine the hours that each light is on and/or dimmed. The maximum target proposed for Part L 2013 compliance for 300 lux and 2,500 hours is 12.8 kWh/m². At the time of writing this had not been confirmed. Refer to CIBSE Society of Light and Lighting website for further details. www.sll.org.uk/resources/partl (accessed 24 March 2013).

31 Refer to **Information Paper 36 – Useful daylight index**.

32 The W/m² allowances are taken from the *BCO Guide to Specification 2009* and were verified by BCO surveys of real buildings. *CIBSE Guide F (Energy Efficiency in Buildings)* adopts similar figures.

33 Data taken from IEA Fact Sheet: *Standby Power Use and the IEA "1-watt Plan"*, April 2007.

34 Refer to **Appendix H** for table of assumptions made for Figures 6.15 and 6.16.

35 It is estimated that data centres use between 1 and 1.5% of global electricity consumption. Source: www1.eere.energy. gov/manufacturing/datacenters/about.html and www.analyticspress.com/datacenters. html. **Appendix H** provides more details on data centre energy consumption.

36 To avoid Legionella risk due to stagnant water, dead legs must be minimised and hot water must be pumped around the domestic hot water circuit. Energy consumption occurs even when hot water is not being used due to the pump energy and heat losses from the pipes.

37 Refer to *The Soft Landings Framework for Better Briefing, Design, Handover and Building Performance In-use* BSRIA BG 4/2009 and www.bsria.co.uk/services/ design/soft-landings.

38 Post-occupancy evaluation is a structured review of a building's performance including occupant satisfaction and energy consumption. Refer to **Appendix H** for further details.

39 The UK's Construction (Design and Management) Regulations 2007 (CDM) state that: 'designers shall in preparing or modifying a design avoid foreseeable risks to the health and safety of any person maintaining the permanent fixtures and fittings of a structure'.

40 The Energy Performance of Buildings (Certificates and Inspections) (England and Wales) Regulations 2007, based on the EU Energy Performance of Buildings (EPDB) Directive, requires inspection of all air conditioning systems with rated outputs over 12 kW at intervals not greater than 5 years. The work must be carried out by an accredited inspector.

41 An analogy is the bus service that wouldn't stop for passengers.

> 'Can any bus service rival the fine Hanley to Bagnall route in Staffordshire? In 1976 it was reported that the buses no longer stopped for passengers. This came to light when one of them, Mr Bill Hancock, complained that buses on the outward journey regularly sailed past queues of up to thirty people. Councillor Arthur Cholerton then made transport history by stating that if these buses stopped to pick up passengers, they would disrupt the time-table.'

The Book of Heroic Failures by Stephen Pile, Futura, 1979.

42 One Planet Living is a global initiative based on ten principles of sustainability. Refer to www.oneplanetliving.org.

CHAPTER 7
Renewable energy

All websites accessed 30 January 2013 unless noted otherwise.

1 A 10% renewables provision in many council planning requirements, often known as the Merton Rule after its first introduction by the Merton Council in London, is inconsistently applied by councils throughout the UK. Some require 10% of energy consumption (kWh) to come from 'renewable or low carbon sources' while others require a 10% reduction in CO_2 emissions. Some councils base the energy/carbon target on the regulated energy in Part L of the Building Regulations, while others include a provision for unregulated energy (small power) to be included in the target. These all lead to different targets, and therefore costs, to developers.

2 Refer to **Appendix L** for further details on the UK Zero Carbon Building and the EU Nearly Zero Energy Building legislation, which are intended to apply to new commercial buildings from 2019 onwards.

3   Data taken from
    www.biomassenergycentre.org.uk,
    www.confusedaboutenergy.co.uk/index.
    php/domestic-fuels/fuel-prices and
    telephone quotes from various energy
    suppliers by the author on 5 November 2012.
    The 10p/kWh electricity tariff used is the day
    rate for a large commercial building. The off-
    peak rate is less than this. Domestic tariffs
    are around 13p/kWh. Detailed time of use
    tariff studies are not included in this book
    and the 10p rate is used throughout.

4   Refer to **Information Paper 30 –
    Government incentives for renewable
    energy** for further details and financial
    implications for Building X and Hotel Y.

5   Data in the British Property Federation/
    Investment Property Databank (BPF/IPD)
    Annual Lease Review 2012, published in
    May 2012, shows that the average office lease
    in the UK in 2011 was less than 8 years.

6   For further details and calculations refer to
    Appendix I.

7   Refer to **Information Paper 23 – Solar hot
    water system types and efficiencies** for
    results from field trials and the difference
    between absorber surface area and gross
    collector area.

8   Refer to **Information Paper 23 – Solar hot
    water system types and efficiencies** for
    example calculation.

9   This is the radiant solar energy from the
    sun falling on 1 m^2 of the earth's surface
    in a year (refer to **Appendix I** for sample
    data). Solar thermal panels are typically
    inclined at around 60° from horizontal
    in London to maximise solar energy
    generation in the winter.

10 The formula for moisture content is
    described in **Appendix I**.

11 Refer to **Appendix I** for values for different
    types of biomass.

12 **Appendix I** contains a worked example
    using unofficial CO_2e emission factors for

biomass to account for black carbon and
life cycle growth of trees.

13 Refer to **Information Paper 25 – Biomass
    and biofuel sources** for further details.

14 The CoP can vary from 5 with a
    temperature difference of 20 °C, to under
    2 when the difference exceeds 60 °C.
    Appendix I provides further details. An
    alternative measure is the system efficiency,
    which is the amount of heat the heat pump
    produces compared to the amount of
    electricity needed to run the entire heating
    system including domestic hot water,
    supplementary heating and pumps. Refer
    also to note 18 for new SCoP legislation.

15 **Appendix I** provides an example calculation
    to illustrate that VRF may potentially
    increase CO_2e emissions compared to
    efficient gas boilers and chillers.

16 *Getting Warmer: A Field Trial of Heat
    Pumps* by the Energy Saving Trust in 2010.
    The Department of Energy and Climate
    Change (DECC) supported the trial and
    noted that: 'Field trials such as these
    are a valuable way of establishing true
    performance in situ, as opposed to in the
    laboratory, and provide useful insights as to
    how performance may be improved'.

17 *A review of Domestic Heat Pump Coefficient
    of Performance* by Iain Staffell (April 2009).

18 The EU Energy Related Products Directive
    2010/30/EU (Supplement No. 626/2011
    dated 4 May 2011) requires, from January
    2013, that manufacturers label the energy
    efficiency of air conditioning systems
    below 12kW using the Seasonal Coefficient
    of Performance (SCOP) for heating and
    the Seasonal Energy Efficiency Ratio
    (SEER) for cooling. There is no correlation
    between the old COP, which measured
    performance at a fixed 7 °C, and the new
    SCOP which calculates the average system
    performance at the variable temperatures
    experienced throughout the heating season
    in three different climate zones. The energy
    consumption in stand-by modes is also
    taken into account. This better reflects real

annual operating conditions. Equipment that was designed to have a peak CoP at 7 °C may not score so highly when running at part heating loads. For example, in northern European climates heat pumps operate at peak load for less than 30% of the time. Minimum standards will tighten in 2014 and consultation is underway to extend the scheme to systems over 12kW.

19 Table 5.10 of the Digest of UK Energy Statistics (DUKES) 2012 states that existing combined cycle gas turbines (CCGT) in the UK had an average thermal to electricity conversion efficiency of 48.5% in 2011. At the new Irsching 4 CCGT plant in Germany, Siemens recorded an efficiency of 60% during testing in May 2011. Available at www.siemens.com/press/en/pressrelease/?press=/en/pressrelease/2011/fossil_power_generation/efp201105064.htm. The efficiency of 55% assumed in Figure 7.10 is therefore probably conservative for new CCGTs in the UK. The electrical distribution losses of 7.5% are taken from clause 5.14 of DUKES 2012.

20 Refer to **Information Paper 24 – Photovoltaic panel types and efficiencies** for an explanation of how solar panels work.

21 Refer to **Information Paper 24 – Photovoltaic panel types and efficiencies**. New solar cells are continually under development, including organic cells, spray-on PV, and cells using graphene and quantum dot technology.

22 Refer to **Information Paper 24 – Photovoltaic panel types and efficiencies** for further calculations.

23 The cost of PV systems has reduced significantly between 2010 and 2012. Refer to **Appendix I** for typical costs of systems in the UK in 2012.

24 Refer to **Information Paper 30 – Government incentives for renewable energy** for the calculation.

25 Refer to **Appendix I**. Outputs are often less than half the design estimates.

26 UK wind farm capacity factors are from Table 6.5 of the Digest of United Kingdom Energy Statistics (DUKES) 2012. In 2010 the capacity factor was only 24% as wind speeds were lower that year. The three previous years saw an average factor of 27%.

27 Refer to **Appendix I** for details on the calculation and assumptions made.

28 Refer to **Appendix I** for cost assumptions.

29 Refer to **Information Paper 27 – Wind turbine performance** for cost data for a selection of commercial wind farms.

30 Refer to **Information Paper 28 – CHP types and efficiencies** for details.

31 The electrical efficiency adopted is 30% which is better than the average efficiency of gas CHP systems in the UK in 2011. The CHP shown in Figure 7.19 could be a 30 kWe unit operating for 1 hour or a 3 kWe unit operating for 10 hours. Refer to **Information Paper 28 – CHP types and efficiencies** for more information on typical CHP efficiencies.

32 The grid electricity factor changes the CO_2e benefit of CHP. In Australia, CHP is always more beneficial (because of the brown and black coal used to produce grid electricity). In France, CHP does not reduce emissions because the grid has a low carbon content (due to the extensive use of nuclear power).

33 *Introducing Combined Heat and Power*, Carbon Trust Technology Guide CTV044, published September 2010.

34 From Tables 7A, 7B and 7C of *DUKES 2012*. Refer also to **Information Paper 28 – CHP types and efficiencies** for a summary of data.

35 Rudolf Diesel hoped that his engines would be more attractive to farmers as they had a source of fuel readily available. In a 1912 presentation to the British Institute of Mechanical Engineers, he stated:

'*The fact that fat oils from vegetable sources can be used may seem insignificant today, but such oils may perhaps become in course of time of the same importance as some natural mineral oils and the tar products are now*'.

One hundred years later his predictions are starting to become reality.

36 Refer to **Appendix B** and **Information Paper 4 – CO_2e emissions from biomass and biofuels** for details on biofuel emission factors.

37 First generation is biofuel from crops. Second generation is biofuel from agricultural residue, industry waste, woody crops, fish oil (leftover gut/waste after fish fillets are produced) and other non-primary food sources. Third generation biofuel generally refers to the production of fuel from algae. Refer to **Information Paper 25 – Biomass and biofuel sources** for further discussion on this.

38 Refer to **Appendix C** for further details and references.

39 Refer to **Appendix L** for more discussion on the cost of carbon.

40 Refer to **Information Paper 30 – UK Government incentives for renewable energy** for further details and financial implications for Building X and Hotel Y.

41 In September 2009, the G20 countries committed to 'rationalize and phase out over the medium term inefficient fossil fuel subsidies that encourage wasteful consumption'. In their *World Energy Outlook 2011*, the International Energy Agency report that 37 governments, which represent half of global fossil-fuel consumption, spent US$409 billion on artificially lowering the price of fossil fuels in 2010, compared to US$66 billion for renewable energy. Only 8% of these subsidies reached the poorest 20% of the population. In the March 2013 budget, the UK government introduced tax breaks for shale gas exploration. A target

for grid electricity decarbonisation will not be set until 2016. The Committee for Climate Change has warned that this raises the possibility of a post-2020 market with little support for renewable technologies. Government incentives are typically needed to help drive industry learning, innovation and cost reduction in renewables.

42 The book can be downloaded free from www.withouthotair.com. It is an excellent and entertaining read and highly recommended.

CHAPTER 8
Lower carbon materials

All websites accessed 30 January 2013 unless noted otherwise.

1 **Appendix J** provides some background on Ecolabels and the EU standard EN 15804 for Environmental Product Declarations released in 2012.

2 Refer to **Information Paper 31 – Embodied carbon of steel versus concrete buildings** for references for these statements.

3 **Appendix J** poses some questions to ask when considering whether to refurbish or replace from a carbon perspective.

4 *Energy and Emission Reduction Opportunities for the Cement Industry*, William T. Choate, US Department of Energy, 29 December 2003.

5 Refer to **Appendix J** for assumptions and calculations. Refer to **Appendix M** for details of Building X.

6 Refer to **Appendix J** for examples.

7 Source: *Sustainable Concrete Architecture* by David Bennett, RIBA Publishing, 2010.

8 Page 9 of *The Procurement and Use of Sustainable Concrete on the Olympic Park, Learning Legacy: Lessons Learned from the*

London 2012 Games Construction Project. Refer to **Appendix J** for ECO$_2$ concrete savings achieved.

9 Refer to **Appendix J** for example calculation. Further information on admixtures is available from www.admixtures.org.uk.

10 *Sustainable Concrete Architecture* (refer to note 7) estimates the ECO$_2$ of reinforcement in the UK to be 0.485 kgCO$_2$e/kg. The Target Zero case studies use 0.82.

11 The University of Bath ICE database gives an ECO$_2$ factor of 5 kgCO$_2$/tonne for general aggregate. *Sustainable concrete Architecture* (refer to note 7) gives the following values (kgCO$_2$/tonne):
   - land-based gravels   8 to 10
   - marine aggregates   negligible
   - crushed rock   20 to 27
   - recycled aggregate   20 to 27
   - china clay stent   20 to 27
   - blast furnace slag   53

12 The estimate of 5% of global emissions in 2004 comes from Section 7.4.5.1 of *Climate Change 2007: Mitigation of Climate Change*, Contribution of Working Group III to the Fourth Assessment Report of the Intergovernmental Panel on Climate Change, 2007. www.ipcc.ch.

13 NovaCem (www.novacem.com) in the UK and TecEco (www.tececo.com) in Australia were developing magnesium oxide cements. In October 2012 Novacem went into liquidation and the company's intellectual property was sold to Australian firm Calix. Research is continuing.

14 Adapted from Energy Fact Sheet, October 2008, World Steel Association. www.worldsteel.org.

15 Refer to **Appendix J** for example ECO$_2$ factors for steel taken from different reference sources.

16 '*The three Rs of sustainable steel*', World Steel Association Fact Sheet, March 2010.

In 2008, more than 475 million tonnes of steel scrap was moved from the waste stream into the recycling stream. The goal for 2050 is 90% recycling, which would result in an additional 38 million tonnes of steel being recycled each year and a saving of 54 million tCO$_2$ compared to steel from raw materials.

17 BRE lifecycle analysis, cited in 'Construction materials report toolkit for carbon neutral developments – Part 1', BioRegional Development Group, 2003. Reproduced in *Reclaimed building Products Guide: A guide to procuring Reclaimed Building Products and Materials* by WRAP.

18 Recycled and reused data taken from the 'Carbon footprint of steel' webpage on Tata Steel website. www.tatasteelconstruction.com/en/sustainability/carbon_and_steel. The waste row in Table 8.5 was added by the author assuming steel that wasn't recycled or reused was sent to waste.

19 Refer to **Appendix J** for further details. For general discussion on the principles of efficient use of metals refer to *Sustainable Materials – With Both Eyes Open* by Allwood et al., UIT Cambridge Ltd, 2012.

20 Refer to **Appendix J** for timber waste data in the UK from TRADA.

21 Refer to note 17.

22 Adapted from *Embodied Carbon: The Inventory of Carbon and Energy (ICE)*, by M. G. Hammond and C. Jones, BSRIA Guide BG10/2011.

23 *Flooring: A Resource Efficiency Action Plan*, WRAP, September 2010. www.wrap.org.uk/sites/files/wrap/Flooring_REAP.pdf.

24 *Carpet Tiles, Learning legacy: Lessons Learned from the London 2012 Games Construction Project.* A case study for the 39,000 m^2 Media Centre showed how the original specification for a bond cut pile tile with a yarn content of 950 g/m^2 was challenged and changed to an Interface

13 Refer to **Information Paper 34 – The green premium – is it real?** for a summary of various studies.

14 Conversation between the author and Miles Keeping, Partner in the real estate team at Deloitte, on 20 November 2012. Refer also to section 10.7 Building value.

15 Taken from Table 3.7a, Annual pay – Gross (£) – For all employee jobs: United Kingdom, 2011, *Annual Survey of Hours and Earnings, 2011 Provisional Results (SOC 2010)*, March 2011, Office for National Statistics. Refer to **Appendix L** for further details.

16 Refer to **Information Paper 33 – Productivity in office buildings** for examples of productivity studies.

17 Adapted from 'Productivity in Buildings: the Killer Variables' by Adrian Leaman and Bill Bordass, in *Creating the Productive Workplace,* 2nd edition, edited by Derek Clements-Croome, E & FN Spon, 2006. Adrian and Bill have been leaders in the measurement of building performance and productivity for over 20 years and established the Usable Buildings Trust in 2002. Refer also to Adrian's presentation at http://www.usablebuildings.co.uk/Pages/Unprotected/KVChicagoApr05.pdf.

18 *A New Era of Sustainability*, UN Global Compact–Accenture CEO Study 2010, June 2010. www.unglobalcompact.org/docs/news_events/8.1/UNGC_Accenture_CEO_Study_2010.pdf.

19 *Faulty Towers: Is the British Office Sustainable* – a report by Gensler, 2006. www.gensler.com/uploads/ documents/da3c78ba84e3e6abe1d04470c8c615b1.pdf.

20 'How going green draws talent, cuts cost' by Dana Mattioli, *The Wall Street Journal*, 13 November 2007. http://online.wsj.com/article/SB119492843191791132.html.

21 *Supply, Demand and the Value of Green Buildings*, Chegut, A., Eichholtz, P. and Kok, N., a Research Report for the Royal Institution of Chartered Surveyors (RICS), March 2012.

22 In a presentation at the BCO Conference in 2012, Philip Irons of Benson Elliot stated that he had interviewed 12 agents and found that sustainability was 'one of the first nice-to-haves that falls away once reality kicks in'. Source: www.architectsjournal.co.uk/footprint/footprint-blog/green-premium-and-brown-discount-do-they-exist/8630939.article. At one of the UK's largest property owners, between 2001 and 2011 not one prospective tenant asked about energy performance prior to signing a lease – refer to **Appendix M**.

23 There have been a number of studies which aim to demonstrate that buildings with good energy ratings or green certification (e.g. BREEAM, LEED, Green Star) have higher value compared to buildings without these. As discussed under higher rents in Section 10.3 Cost of occupancy, there are some concerns regarding the sample sizes and reliability of the results and these should be treated with caution. Refer to **Information Paper 34 – The green premium – is it real?** for examples of studies.

24 Refer to note 18.

25 *Insights into Climate Change Adaptation by UK Companies*, a report prepared for DEFRA by the Carbon Disclosure Project, March 2012.

26 Refer to **Information Paper 2 – Adapting buildings to climate change**.

27 The energy supply to buildings is not infallible, with fuel shortages and power outages occurring for various reasons – natural disasters, political leverage and lack of investment in ageing infrastructure. While these are national issues, how well a building copes in such scenarios could be considered a risk to business continuity.

28 www.utm.edu/staff/jfieser/vita/research/busbook.htm.

29 The press release dated 3 August 2012 from the Investment Management Association stated total funds under management by their members in Q2, 2012 as £598 billion with ethical funds accounting for £6.9 billion of this total. www.investmentuk.org/press-centre/2012/press-release-statisticsq212/.

30 *Climate Impact Reporting for Property Investment Portfolios: A Guide for Pension Funds and Their Trustees and Fund Managers*, Institutional Investors Group on Climate Change (IIGCC), 2010.

31 The Carbon Trust guide CTV067 *Making the Business Case for a Carbon Reduction Project: How to Win Over the Board and Influence People* provides advice to energy/environmental managers, facilities managers and engineers on how to present projects to decision makers to give them the best chance of obtaining approval and implementation. www.carbontrust.com/media/169595/j7896_ctv067_making_the_business_case_for_03.pdf.

32 Various studies have shown that there is a discrepancy between the perceived cost and actual cost of greener buildings in the industry:
  - -0.4 to 12.5% – cost premium for green buildings (actual costs based on various studies)
  - 0.9 to 29% – estimated cost premium for green buildings (based on design stage estimates and surveys).
  For further details refer to *The Business Case for Green Building: A Review of the Costs and Benefits for Developers, Investors and Occupants*, World Green Building Council, 2013. www.worldgbc.org.

In conclusion

1 Urban areas tend to get warmer than rural areas due to the extensive use of surface materials such as concrete and asphalt, which effectively retain heat, and the lack of vegetation (which provides cooling through evapotranspiration). Methods of mitigation include lighter coloured surfaces to reflect heat and green roofs.

2 At a supermarket in North East England the 'turn off lights to save energy' stickers in the back of house areas were not getting much traction with staff. When these were changed to 'saving energy increases your bonus' the results were very different. Staff even started researching lighting technologies and making suggestions to management on how to cut energy further.

3 The first LED backlit LCD TV, the Qualia KDX46Q005, was introduced by Sony in August 2004 and cost US$10,000. Eight years later, due to improvements in manufacturing processes and fierce competition, a 46 inch LED TV now costs under US$1,000. Source: http://en.wikipedia.org/wiki/Qualia_(Sony) and www.amazon.com Accessed on 30 January 2013.

Acknowledgements

This book would not have been possible without the generosity and support of a lot of people. I would like to thank the following, and if I have missed anyone out please forgive me (and I'll buy you a beer):

- The partners at Cundall for indulging me in writing the book and allowing me to use work resources for research.
- The team of reviewers who waded through the first drafts and provided comments, corrections and encouragement: Rhodri Evans (Balfour Beatty), Ania Hampton (Hampton Consulting), Daniel Winder (Sheppard Robson), Prof. Angus McIntosh (Real Estate Forecasting Ltd), and from Cundall, Andrew Thompson, Jack Devlin, Stephen Maddocks, Andrew Moore and Robert van Zyl.
- Cundall partners and staff who provided comments on specific topics including: Peter O'Halloran (building services), Andrew Bissell (lighting), Simon Wyatt (renewables), Gavin Clifford (structural), Geoff Carter (civil), Tania Clark (transport) and Andrew Parkin (acoustics).
- The following, who generously shared data or provided comments on specific topics:
    - operating carbon – Chris Botten (Better Buildings Partnership) and Bill Bordass (Usable Buildings Trust)
    - embodied carbon – Dr Craig Jones (Sustain), Kristian Steele (Arup) and Andrew Minson (Concrete Centre).
    - business case – Miles Keeping (Deloitte).
- Gemma Dawson (book) and Hayley Bone (appendices) for turning my doodles into coherent diagrams and illustrations.
- The team at RIBA Publishing who never lost enthusiasm despite the manuscript being over a year late: Lucy, Sharon, Matthew, Kate, Alex, Andy and Steven.
- Caimin McCabe and Alan Fogarty of Cundall for sharing ideas, technical advice and interesting debates over the past 8 years. Much appreciated.
- Dr Graham Treloar of Deakin University for his pioneering work in embodied carbon in the early 2000s – a good bloke, sadly missed.

Any errors, omissions and misplaced opinions still remaining, despite the best efforts of the above, are entirely my own.

Finally, I would like to thank Alison, Laura and Katie for putting up with late nights and endless weekends sat at the laptop. Sorry!

Photograph credits

		Credit	Building
	Intro	Tim Soar www.valencyarchive.co.uk	The Tea Building, London
	Part 1	Tim Soar www.valencyarchive.co.uk	One Wood Street, London
	Chapter 1	Yang Qitao / HASSELL www.hassellstudio.com	HASSELL Studio, Shanghai
	Chapter 2	Tim Soar www.valencyarchive.co.uk	24 Britton Street, London
	Chapter 3	Great Portland Estates	180 Great Portland Street, London
	Chapter 4	Adrian Roche Cundall	Cannon Place, London
	Chapter 5	Martine Hamilton Knight www.builtvision.co.uk	Waverley Court, City of Edinburgh Council HQ
	Part 2	Mark Waugh www.markwaugh.net	Fabrica, Manchester
	Chapter 6	BIM model by Cundall	Snowhill 2, Birmingham
	Chapter 7	Jonathan Miller www.jmillerphotography.com	Westfield Sydney City
	Chapter 8	Kristen McCluskie www.kristenmccluskie.com	Palatine Centre, University of Durham
	Chapter 9	Kristen McCluskie www.kristenmccluskie.com	Harton Technology College, South Shields
	Chapter 10	Kristen McCluskie www.kristenmccluskie.com	Grey Group fitout, The Johnson Building, London
	Conclusion	Morley von Sternberg www.vonsternberg.com	Basepoint Business and Innovation Centre, Luton

Glossary

TERM	DEFINITION
base building	The common areas and services of an office building provided by the landlord.
BIM	Building Information Modelling – a detailed 3D model of a building including data on all of the components (materials, product details, etc.).
black carbon	Soot and particulates from the incomplete combustion of fossil fuels and biomass which contributes to global warming. Refer to Appendix B.
BREEAM	Building Research Establishment Environmental Assessment Method – an environmental rating tool for buildings in the UK. International versions are also available.
Btu	British Thermal Units – a measure of energy consumption. Refer to Appendix A for conversion factor to kWh.
calorific value	The amount of energy in a fuel (kWh per quantity of fuel). Refer to Appendix B for explanation of gross CV and net CV.
CO_2	Carbon dioxide – the main greenhouse gas contributing to global warming. Refer to Appendix A.
CO_2e	Carbon dioxide equivalent – the combined global warming potential of the three main greenhouse gases: CO_2, methane (CH_4) and nitrous oxide (N_2O).
CoP	Coefficient of Performance – the efficiency of heat pumps in turning electricity into heat.
CSR	Corporate social responsibility – usually relates to reporting of environmental and social performance.
DEC	Display Energy Certificate – an operating energy rating tool in the UK.
DGNB	The German Green Building Council's environmental rating tool for buildings.
DHW	Domestic hot water.
discount rate	The rate used to convert future cash flows into present values taking into account inflation, cost of borrowing and investment risk. A value of 5% has been adopted in this book.
ECO_2	An abbreviation for embodied carbon.
embodied carbon	The CO_2e emissions due to the energy consumed in manufacturing, delivering and installing the materials used to build, refurbish and fit-out a building, and their disposal at end of life. Also includes the CO_2 emissions from chemical reactions in material production.
Energy Star	An operating energy rating tool in the USA.
EPC	Energy Performance Certificate – a design energy rating tool in the UK. Different versions are used in other European countries.
F-gas	Fluorinated gases are potent greenhouse gases and included in the UNFCCC. Refer to Appendix B for emission factors.
GHG	Greenhouse gases – carbon dioxide, methane, nitrous oxide plus the three F-gases. Refer to Appendix A.
GIA	Gross internal area. The floor area of a building measured to the internal face of the perimeter walls at each floor level.

TERM	DEFINITION
Green Star	An environmental rating tool for buildings in Australia.
HVAC	Heating, ventilation and cooling building services.
IPCC	Intergovernmental Panel on Climate Change.
kWh	Kilowatt-hours – a measure of energy consumption which can be used for primary energy, electricity, fossil fuel, heating and cooling.
LEED	Leadership in Energy and Environmental Design. An environmental rating tool for buildings in the USA and internationally.
Lux level	The amount of light reaching a surface measured in lumens per m^2.
mixed mode	A ventilation system which uses a combination of natural and mechanical ventilation.
MJ	Megajoules – a measure of energy consumption. Refer to Appendix A for conversion factor to kWh.
NABERS	National Australian Building Environmental Rating Scheme – a rating tool for operating energy, water and waste in buildings.
net present cost	The difference between the present value of the future cash flows from an investment and the amount of investment. A discount rate is used to convert future cash flows into net present values.
NLA	Net Lettable Area – the area leased by the tenants. This is typically the GIA less toilets, lift, plant rooms, stairs, lift wells, common entrance halls, lobbies, corridors, internal structural walls and car parking areas.
oGIA	Occupied Gross Internal Area – a unit of floor area in m^2 used in this book for benchmarking energy consumption. Refer to Appendix D. oGIA = GIA × occupied NLA/total NLA
operating carbon	The CO_2e emissions due to the consumption of electricity, gas and other fuels used in a building for heating, cooling, ventilation, lighting, hot water, computers, servers and other equipment.
Part L	The conservation of fuel and power component of the UK Building Regulations (2010 version unless noted otherwise).
primary energy	The energy in a fuel source in its natural state before being converted to a secondary form of energy such as electricity. Refer to Appendix A for conversion factors.
radiative forcing	The heating (or cooling) of the climate due to anthropogenic (man-made) and natural factors. Refer to Appendix A.
regulated energy	The energy consumption covered by Part L of the Building Regulations which typically includes fixed building services, heating, hot water, cooling, ventilation and lighting.
SCoP	Seasonal Coefficient of Performance – the average annual CoP of a heat pump in a particular climate zone.
toe	Tonnes of oil equivalent – a measure of energy consumption. Refer to Appendix A for conversion factor to kWh.
transport carbon	The CO_2e emissions due to the energy used by people commuting to and from a building.
UNFCCC	United Nations Framework Convention on Climate Change.
unregulated energy	The energy consumption in a building not covered by Part L of the Building Regulations. This may include small power, lifts, special equipment and external lighting.

Index

About the author

David Clark has over 20 years' experience designing buildings in the UK and Australia, is chartered in both structural and building services engineering, and has specialised in sustainability since 2002. He was the principal author of the first Green Star rating tool in Australia and has worked on numerous award-winning green buildings. David is a Partner with Cundall Johnston & Partners and, in addition to working on building designs, leads their corporate sustainability and R&D activities.

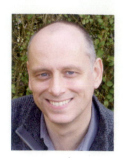

About Cundall

Cundall Johnston & Partners LLP ("Cundall") is a multi-disciplinary engineering design practice with offices in the UK, Europe, MENA, Asia and Australia. They have a strong reputation for the sustainable design and analysis of buildings which is recognised through numerous awards. Cundall was the first consultancy to be endorsed as a One Planet Company by BioRegional. For further details on their services, projects and office locations, and to contact the author, refer to **www.cundall.com**.

AUTHOR ROYALTIES

This book was not written to make money. All of the author royalties are paid to Cundall Johnston & Partners LLP who will then distribute annually as follows:

- 30% to protect amazon rainforest via Cool Earth (www.coolearth.org).
- 30% to environmental and social charities nominated by the Cundall Sustainability Committee.
- 40% to the Cundall Innovation Fund to support R&D activities for a sustainable built environment.

Author photo by Katie McCaig-Clark